NEONATAL BACTERIAL INFECTION

Edited by **Bernhard Resch**

Neonatal Bacterial Infection
http://dx.doi.org/10.5772/3317
Edited by Bernhard Resch

Contributors

Ketevan Nemsadze, Friedrich Reiterer, Ursula Kiechl-Kohlendorfer, Elke Griesmaier, Nora Hofer, Wilhelm Müller, Bernhard Resch, Christina Cimenti, Wolfgang Erwa, Wilhelm Müller, Bernhard Resch, Elisabeth Resch, Bernhard Resch

Published by InTech

Janeza Trdine 9, 51000 Rijeka, Croatia

Publishing Process Manager Sandra Bakic
Technical Editor InTech DTP team
Cover InTech Design team

Additional hard copies can be obtained from orders@intechopen.com

Neonatal Bacterial Infection, Edited by Bernhard Resch
p. cm.
ISBN 978-953-51-1124-5

For EU product safety concerns:
IN TECH d.o.o., Prolaz Marije Krucifikse Kozulić 3, 51000 Rijeka, Croatia,
info@intechopen.com or visit our website at intechopen.com.

Meet the editor

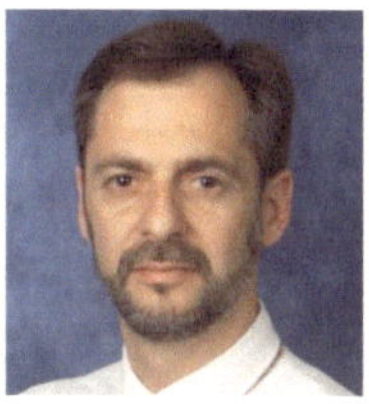

Born in Graz, Austria, Prof. Bernhard Resch received his medical degree at the Karl – Franzens University Graz in 1988. Following post-doc studies at the Division of Neonatology, and the Department of Pediatric Surgery of the University Hospital Graz, he became consultant of Pediatrics in 1997 and consultant of Neonatal and Pediatric Intensive Care Medicine in 2000. In 2004 he became Associate Professor of Pediatrics and in 2008 Head of the Research Unit of Neonatal Infectious Diseases and Epidemiology of the Medical University Graz. In 2012 he became Professor of Pediatrics. His main research fields include neonatal infectious diseases, respiratory syncytial virus infection, and periventricular leukomalacia of the preterm infant.He is member and board member of several national and international scientific societies; currently he is president of the Austrian Society of Perinatal Medicine, and member of the editorial board of several international journals including The Open Microbiology Journal and Journal of Neonatal Biology. Prof. Resch is married and has four children between 13 and 23 years of age.

Contents

Preface

Neonatal bacterial infection and sepsis are clinical syndromes characterized by systemic signs of infection associated with bacteraemia within the first month of life. There are two patterns of disease with different spectrums of causative agents, early- and late-onset sepsis. Neonatal sepsis still remains a significant cause of morbidity and mortality in the newborn, particularly in preterm, low birth weight infants [Stoll and Hansen 2003]. Despite advances in neonatal care, overall case-fatality rates from sepsis range from 3% to as high as 50% [Palazzi 2001]. Clinical signs of bacterial infection are vague and non-specific, and up to now there exists no easily available, reliable marker of infection despite a large bulk of studies focussing on inflammatory indices in neonatology.

Bacterial pathogens that cause neonatal infections include Group-B-Streptococci (GBS), Escherichia coli, Haemophilus influenzae, Enterococci, Listeria monozytogenes, Streptococcus viridans, Streptococcus pneumoniae, and Staphylococcus aureus as the most common ones for early-onset infections and coagulase-negative Staphylococci (CONS), E.coli, Enterococci, Klebsiella pneumoniae, Staphylococcus aureus, and Streptococcus viridans for late-onset infections. The identity of each may be suggested by timing of infection, presentation of signs and symptoms, and response to empirically prescribed antibiotics. For all organisms, successful management requires thorough, thoughtful assessment of risk factors, complete and careful clinical and laboratory studies, and prompt initiation of antibiotics and supportive treatment.

Every neonatologist is faced with the uncertainty of under- or over- diagnosing bacterial infection, and positive blood cultures are not the "philosopher´s stone" per se. As a result many neonates and especially those born preterm receive empiric antibiotic therapy, and the longer they are treated the more resistant pathogens develop in case of unconfirmed infection. If the clinical picture combined with a negative culture result allows justification of the neonate as being not infected antibiotics should be terminated as early as possible.

In this book three topics will be discussed: clinical presentation including a general approach to "sepsis neonatorum" and two distinct diagnoses – pneumonia and osteomyelitis – diagnostic approaches including C-reactive protein and the immature myeloid information, and prevention and treatment of bacterial infection with immunoglobulins.

Bernhard Resch, MD
Research Unit for Neonatal Infectious Diseases and Epidemiology,
Medical University of Graz, Austria
Division of Neonatology, Department of Pediatrics, Graz,
Austria

Section 1

Clinical Presentation

Chapter 1

Early Detection and Prevention of Neonatal Sepsis

Ketevan Nemsadze

Additional information is available at the end of the chapter

http://dx.doi.org/10.5772/56121

1. Introduction

Sepsis has been a burden to mankind for millions of years and will continue to plague man as long as microorganisms exist here on earth. Only recently the medical community has started celebrating the World Sepsis Day (WSD) which was established in 2012, yet a decade before, at the end of the 20th century the Anti-Sepsis Center was founded in Georgia. [1]

Research shows that early recognition and intervention saves lives. To achieve this improvement requires a partnership between the public, parents, and healthcare professions. Sepsis is a common pediatric problem. Severe sepsis and septic shock are among the leading causes of death in infants and have an overall pediatric mortality rate of 8-10%. Definitive diagnosis requires clinical identification of infection in a patient who also meets the clinical criteria for the Systemic Inflammatory Response Syndrome (SIRS). [2]

In the given chapter, early recognition, diagnostic criteria, treatment and prevention of neonatal sepsis are described.

2. Definition

Neonatal Sepsis – is a clinical syndrome which is a general reaction to infection. Neonatal sepsis is characterized by systemic inflammation and general damage of tissues. Clinical definition is based on existing infection and systemic inflammatory response. Neonatal sepsis is diagnosed on the basis of clinical or microbiological data. Neonatal sepsis is an irreversible process which may cause mortality in cases of untimely detection and treatment. [3]

3. Terminology

Frequently Used Terms Referring to Sepsis: Neonatal Fever; Neonatal Sepsis; Serious Bacterial Infection (SBI); Systemic Inflammatory Response Syndrome (SIRS); Septic Shock (= Sepsis + Cardiovascular dysfunction).[2]

Classifications of Neonatal Sepsis

Neonatal and infant sepsis is classified according to age at the time of disease manifestation.

'EARLY' SEPSIS_manifests within the first 72 hours after birth by the vertical transfer of microorganisms existing in maternal passages. It is characterized by fulminant multiple organ damage. Symptoms of pneumonia may be revealed within the first week of life.

'EARLY, EARLY' SEPSIS AND VERY EARLY SEPSIS manifests within the first 24 hours after birth by the vertical transfer of microorganisms existing in maternal passages.

'LATE' SEPSIS manifests within the first 72 hours after birth by the vertical or horizontal transfer of microorganisms existing in maternal passages. The primary cause of late sepsis is hospital infection. It is characterized by gradual development and multiple nidus of infection. Meningitis can occur quite frequently. Sepsis may manifest within the first 3 months of the child's life.

LATE, LATE' SEPSIS OR VERY LATE SEPSIS manifests more than 3 months after birth mainly in children born before 28 weeks of pregnancy or with immunodeficiency.[4,3]

Frequency of Early Sepsis of Neonates (Tbilisi Central Children's hospital)

Full-Term Infants: 0.2% (among 2/1000 neonates)

Late pre-term infant: 0.3% (among 3/1000 neonates)

Low Birth-Weight Infants: 1.5% (15/1000 neonates)

Very Low Birth-Weight Infants: 2.5% (25/1000 neonates)

Extremely Low Birth-Weight Infants: 25% (250/1000 neonates)

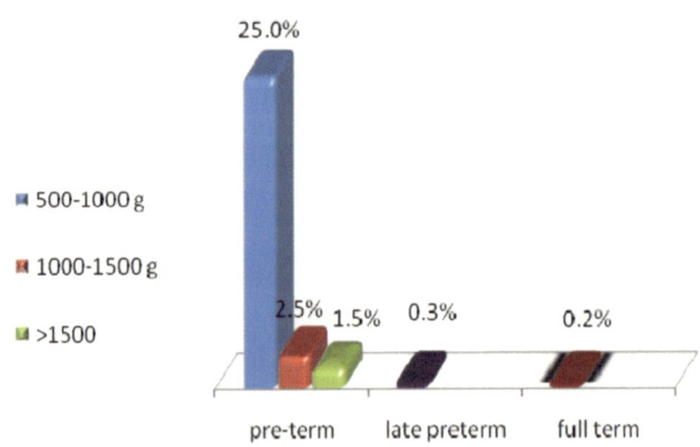

Figure 1. K. Nemsadze, Neonatology, 2010 [1]

The frequency of early sepsis in infants with extremely low-birth-weight is 100 times higher than in full-term babies. Considering the fact that the number of children born at a gestational age greater than 35 weeks is much more common, the data shows that neonates with low birth weight are far more likely to be diagnosed with sepsis. [1]

Frequency of Late Sepsis of Neonates

Late Sepsis is predominantly nosocomial (hospital disease) thought in some cases infection may be connected with maternal organisms. This form of clinical sepsis is one of main clinical problems characterized primarily by significantly premature babies. Development of late sepsis in neonates of this group is associated with a significant increase in the frequency of complications, mortality and the prolonged hospitalization of neonates.

In West Europe, North America and Australia – late sepsis frequency is up to 6 among 1000 neonates. Among neonates of gestational age less of 25 weeks, late sepsis develops in 46% of them; among neonates of gestational age between 25-28 weeks, late sepsis develops in 29%. Thus, the less gestational age the higher the probability of developing late sepsis. The frequency of nosocomial infections is inversely proportional to birth weight and gestational age of neonates. This complication cannot only be explained by the prolonged hospitalization needs of extremely premature children. [5]

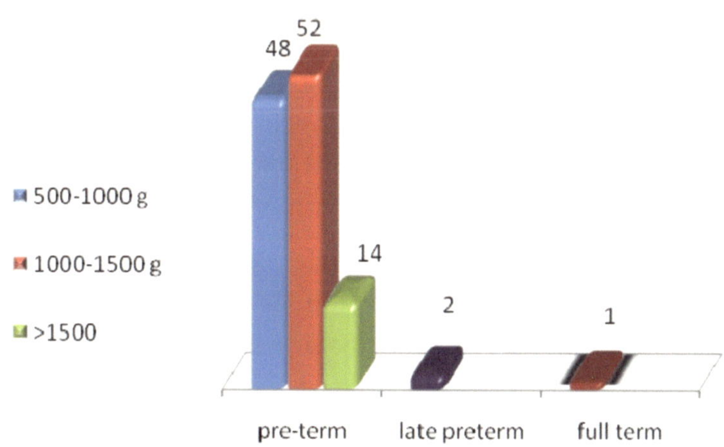

Figure 2. K. Nemsadze, Neonatology, 2010 [1]

4. Etiology and epidemiology

Etiological Structure of Sepsis in Developed Countries

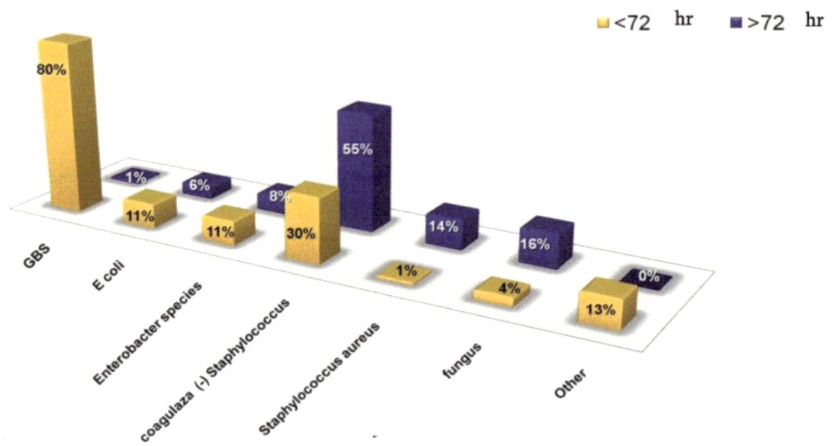

Figure 3. J. Garcia-Prats et al.,SeminPediatrInfect Dis, 2000;11:4 [6]

Etiological Structure of Sepsis in Tbilisi Children's Central Hospital

Consequently, the main causative agents of neonatal sepsis are bacteria such as staphylococcus.

Klebsiella, acinetobacter and staphylococcus aureus can be the cause of early as well as late sepsis

Late sepsis is usually a nosocomial disease although is some cases it may be connected with vertical infection. Pseudomonas, salmonella and serratia can often cause late sepsis. Many factors impact the etiological structure, including the quality of life, cultural traditions, practice of antibiotic therapy and the possibility of distorted results caused by many neonates to die at home.

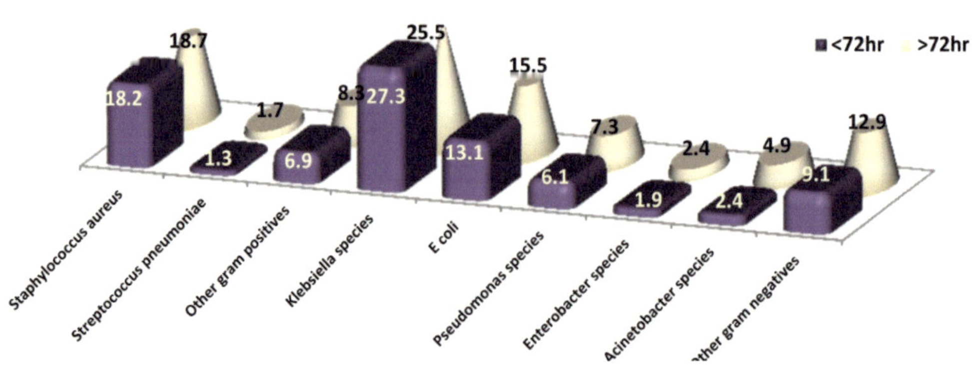

Figure 4. K. Nemsadze, Neonatology, 2010 [1]

5. Pathophysiology

In the presence of sepsis, the response of infection released anti-inflammatory mediators can't localize anti-inflammatory process. Generalized infection is formed as sepsis. The cause of sepsis (SIRS) is multi-factorial: Activation of anti-inflammatory mediators; complement ischemia of tissues; cytopathology; changes in apoptosis rate. Cellular damage with discharge of anti-inflammators (IL1, IL6 TNF- Tumor Necrosis Factor) and anti-inflammatory mediators increase the probability of developing multi-organ failure. The cardiovascular system, pulmonary system, gastro-intestinal tract, kidneys and neurological system are most frequently damaged. Given mediators stimulate production of various proteins called as reagents of acute phase. Any kinds of inflammation stimulus, including infection, trauma and ischemia causes marginal extravasations and activation of granulocytes and monocytes with the simultaneous release of anti-inflammatory cytokines including interleukins IL1, IL6 TNF (Tumor Necrosis Factor) [7]

Sepsis is caused by Systemic Inflammatory Response (SIR)

It is widely known that sepsis educes as a result of Systemic Inflammatory Response (SIR). In the process of opsonization and macrophage phagocytosis pathogens cause the formation of various anti-inflammatory mediators (cytokines) which damage vessel endothelium the result of which is the release of tissue factors. The coagulation system is activated and fibrinolysis inhibitor activity is increased. [8,9]

Anti-inflammatory Mediators are Reagents of the Acute Phase

After the patient is stabilized, normalization and a secondary increase in the levels of CBC indicate the sepsis complication (*subdural empyema and bacterial meningitis* [10]. Sepsis may change the metabolism of neonates. The change in metabolism may be described in two phases

Ebb Phase → Flow Phase

EBB Phase

The initial EBB phase lasts 1-3 days. In this phase the neonate is at the stage of compensation while metabolism is slowed.

EBB Phase Consists of Some Clinical Symptoms:

- Hypometabolism
- Decrease of energy consumption
- Reduction of cardiac output
- Hypoxia
- Vasoconstriction

Flow Phase

Flow Phase follows the initial Ebb Phase. In this phase the organism goes into a hyperactive state, which is particularly conditioned by a hyper inflammatory reaction. In many cases flow phase leads to patient mortality.

Flow Phase Includes Some Clinical Symptoms:

- Hypermetabolism
- Increase in energy consumption
- Increase in cardiac output
- Hyperoxia

6. Risk factors

Maternal Premature Birth Risk Factors

- Preterm rupture of the fetus membrane
- Anhydrous periodgreater than 18 hours
- Febrile temperature greater than38°C (at or after birth)
- GBS bacteriuria during current pregnancy (>104 cfu/mL)
- GBS bacterial colonization of the vagina/perineum
- Chorioamnionitis/Endometritis
- Infection of the Urino-Genital Systems
- Invasive Procedures
- Previous child with GBS infection
- Previous child born with sepsis
- Multiple pregnancy

Neonatal Risk Factors

- Premature neonate less than 37 weeks of gestation, Low birth weight and Small for Gestational Age(SGA)
- Male sex
- Stable intranatal fetal tachycardia
- Asphyxia/Resuscitation
- Hypothermia
- Invasive procedures
- Artificial feeding
- Non-insurance fetus
- Lack of "Skin-to-skin" contact with mother
- Long-term Hospitalization; Irrational antibiotic therapy
- Poor sanitary habits of medical personnel.

It is essential to know the evidence-based risk factors of neonatal infection as modern strategies of prophylaxis are precisely based on this data. [11]

Change of Body Temperature as a Sign of Possible Infection in Neonates

The use of a mercury glass thermometer is considered the gold standard for measuring the normal body temperature of neonates – 36.5 – 37.5 C. Sepsis is characterized by arise in temperature or hypothermia. Rise of temperature greater than38°C that lasts more than an hour is associated with infection process.[12]

On the analysis of their research, Klein and Marcy made the following conclusions referring to diagnostic analysis of symptoms and the relation to rising body temperature in full-term neonates: If bodily temperature is less than 38 °C, 99.9% of neonates will not develop sepsis. When among neonates with body temperature more than 38 °C, only 10% are expected to developed sepsis.

7. Clinical symptomatology

Nonspecific clinical signs: (3P-Signs)

- Poor breathing
- Poor sucking
- Poor looking

Clinical signs are various and the diversity of symptoms is the result of metabolic and inflammatory processes arisen in case of neonatal sepsis. [12]

Consequently, clinical symptoms of sepsis are nonspecific: They cannot be summarized according to principles: Poor Breathing, Poor Eating and Poor Looking. Out of 10 children with suspected sepsis, the disease will be confirmed in only one.

Symptoms of Respiratory Disorders:

- Tachypnea (>60 in min)
- Chest retraction
- Grunting while breathing
- Inflating the nostrils (nose wings)
- Apnea/bradypnea (<30 in a min)
- Hypoxia
- Irregular breathing [12]

Symptoms of Gastro-intestinal and Neurologic Disorders:

- Gastro-intestinal
- Loss of appetite
- Vomiting; Diarrhea
- Abdominal distension
- Splenomegaly
- Neurologic
- Convulsions
- Hypotonia and Hypodynamia
- Lethargy [12]

Symptoms of Cardiovascular and Skin Disorders:

Cardiovascular:

- Hypotension

- Metabolic Acidosis
- Tachycardia

Skin:

- Pale or marble with petechia or purple
- Mottling
- Cold or wet
- Cyanosis
- Jaundice [12]

8. Evaluations criteria of neonatal sepsis

Bacterial inoculation of blood; Leukocytes (<5 or >30x10^9/l); Total number of neutrophils; Leukocyte index (LI) >0,2; CRP >10 mg/l (Initial examination no later than 12 hours from birth); ESR > 15 mm/hr; Chest X-ray in the presence of Respiratory Distress Syndrome (RDS); Lumbar puncture in the presence of neurological symptoms; Bacterial inoculation of urine by using catheter or suprapubic puncture. [13]

Lumbar Puncture (LP): When should *a lumbar puncture be conducted?*

Symptoms of sepsis and any of the following symptoms;

Bulging of fontanel, any neurological symptoms, leukocytes < 5 or > 30 x 109 in 24 hours or > 20 x 109 since second 24 hours or Leukocyte Index (LI) > 0,4 or CRP > 40 mg/l or> 2, laboratory Indexes with obvious abnormality.[13]

Evaluation Criteria of Late Sepsis

Common clinical conditions if sepsis is suspected; Instability of body temperature; Gastro-intestinal symptoms (vomiting, abdominal distension, blood in stool, increase in quantity of residual mass in stomach); Neurological symptoms; Cardiorespiratory dysfunction (100<HR> 180, 30
 60, hypotension, time of capillary filling > 4 sec); Respiratory symptoms (toughening of parameters of lungs mechanical ventilation of BR > 60, apnoea); Metabolic acidosis; hyperglycemia/hypoglycemia; Leukocytosis; leukopenia; Ratio of immature neutrophils compared to the total number of neutrophils (LI)>2,0 , thrombocytopenia

Treatment should starts in case of possible sepsis if;the mother is suspected of having infection; the infant has clinical signs of infection; the infant has possible signs of infection in combination with low weight at birth, asphyxia and other risk factors; positive results of screening tests and/or bacterial investigation.

9. Indication of prophylaxis usage of antibiotics during delivery

GBS bacteruria during pregnancy; Previous child with GBS infection; Mother's temperature greater than 38°C, even when GBS culture is negative; Unknown GBS status and early discharge of amniotic fluid >18 hr., gestational age less than 37 weeks, mother's temperature is greater than 38°C. [2]

Antenatal Prophylaxis

It is important to use a wide variety of laboratory methods for identification of GBS (Group B streptococcus). Defining the number of colonies in urine of pregnant women is necessary to diagnose GBS.[2]

Main changes in the 2010 guidelines include the following: Intranatal Prophylaxis - Change of penicillin-G recommended dose for chemoprophylaxis; Updating schemes of prophylaxis for women with an allergy to penicillin and revising the algorithms. [2]

Secondary Prophylaxis of GBS in Case of Early Sepsis of Neonates

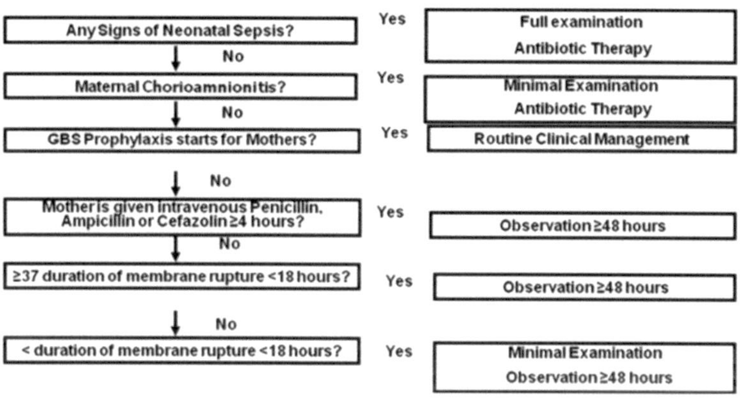

Figure 5. Prevention of Perinatal Group B Streptococcal Disease Revised Guidelines from CDC, 2010 [11]

Full diagnostic evaluation includes a blood culture, a complete blood count (CBC) including white blood cell differential and platelet counts, chest radiograph (if respiratory abnormalities are present), and lumbar puncture (if patient is stable enough to tolerate procedure and sepsis is suspected).Antibiotic therapy should be directed toward the most common causes of neonatal sepsis, including intravenous ampicillin for GBS and coverage for other organisms (including Escherichia coli and other gram-negative pathogens) and should take into account local antibiotic resistance patterns. Consultation with obstetric providers is important to determine the level of clinical suspicion for chorioamnionitis. Chorioamnionitis is diagnosed clinically and some of the signs are nonspecific. Limited evaluation includes blood culture (at birth) and CBC with differential and platelets (at birth and/or at 6–12 hours of life). If signs of sepsis develop, a full diagnostic evaluation should be conducted and antibiotic therapy initiated. If 37 weeks' gestation, observation may occur at home after 24 hours if other discharge criteria have been met, access to medical care is readily available and a person who is able to comply fully with instructions for home observation will be present. If any of these conditions are not met, the infant should be observed in the hospital for at least 48 hours and until discharge criteria are achieved. Some experts recommend a CBC with differential and platelets at age 6–12 hours. [11]

10. Principles of treatment

Early Sepsis – Ampicillin + Gentamicin; Late Sepsis – Cefotaxime+ Aminoglycosides; Consequent A/B therapy depending on the results of repeated blood inoculation - Vancomycin and/or Meropenem and/or Antimycotic Drugs.

It's important to consider local epidemiological/microbiological data.

Empyreal antibiotic therapy of early sepsis must impact on gram negative and gram positive microorganisms. It's important to remember that listerias are potential agents for early infection of neonates. It is necessary to prescribe 2 antibiotics which cover a wide enough spectrum and at the same time resist a selection of antibiotic resistant bacteria. In case of late hospital sepsis it is particularly important to affect staphylococcus and gram negative bacteria. If mother discharges GBS during delivery it is advised that penicillin be prescribed.

NB! Cephalosporin is ineffective towards enterococcus and listerias!

Figure 6. Therapeutic guidelines in neonatal infection 2011[11]

Duration of Antibacterial Therapy

Absence of clinical symptoms and negative results of investigation: 48-72 hr; In case of gram + flora – 7 or more days; In case of gram + flora - minimum 14 days; In case of meningitis - 21 days; Consequent a/b therapy should depend on the results of repeated blood culture investigations.[12]

The duration of antibacterial therapy depends on clinical form of infection while therapy of osteomyelitis/endocarditis it is recommended to change antibiotics only in case of absence of effect of conducted therapy.

Dosage of Antibiotics: Ampicilin

AMPICILIN - Single dose 25-50 mg/kg IntraV/IntraM GBS Infection.

In cases of bacteria it is permitted- 150-200 mg/kg/day;

In cases of meningitis- 300- 400 mg/kg in a day

Gestational Age (weeks.)	Child Age (days)	Interval between Injection (hours)
≤ 29	0-28	12
	> 28	8
30-36	0-14	12
	> 14	8
37-44	0-7	12
	> 7	8
≥ 45	All	6

Table 1. Therapeutic guidelines in neonatal infection 2011 [11]
Neofax 2009 Twenty Second Edition [14]

Dosage of Antibiotics: Gentamicin

GENTAMICIN

Injected intravenously slowly during 30 minutes.

Gestational Age (weeks.)	Postnatal Age (days)	Dose (mg/kg)	Interval between Injection (hours)
≤ 29	0-7	5	48
	8-28	4	34
	≥ 29	4	24
30-34	0-7	4,5	36
	≥ 8	4	24
≥ 35	All	4	24

Table 2. Therapeutic guidelines in neonatal infection 2011 [11]
Neofax 2009 Twenty Second Edition [14]

Dosage of Antibiotics: Amikacin

AMIKACIN

Injected intravenously slowly during 30 minutes.

Gestational Age (weeks.)	Postnatal Age (days)	Dose (mg/kg)	Interval between Injection (hours)
≤ 29	0-7	18	48
	8-28	15	36
	≥ 29	15	24
30-34	0-7	18	36
	≥ 8	15	24
≥ 35	All	15	24

Table 3. Therapeutic guidelines in neonatal infection 2011 [11]
Neofax 2009 Twenty Second Edition [14,15]

Dosage of Antibiotics: Cefotaxime

CEFOTAXIME

Single Dose 50 mg/kg intravenously slowly during 30 minutes *Or I/M*

The dosage of antibiotics is relevant to the etiological agent and depends on gestational and postnatal age of the neonate and it is chosen according to the Neofax guide.[14]

Gestational Age (weeks.)	Postnatal Age (days)	Interval between Injection (hours)
≤ 29	0-28 > 28	12 8
30-36	0-14 > 14	12 8
37-44	0-7 > 7	12 8
≥ 45	All	6

Table 4. Therapeutic guidelines in neonatal infection 2011[11]
Neofax 2009 Twenty Second Edition [14]

11. Consultation with parents

Complications include the following: Septic shock; Necrotic tonsillitis enterocolitis, ulcero-necrotic enterocolitis; Subdural empyema; Meningitis

Information for Patients

What is Sepsis?

Sepsis – Is the existence of infection in the blood. Sepsis is a serious disease that impacts the whole body. Treatment of Sepsis should be started immediately after diagnosis, because the late start of treatment may endanger life. Sepsis may occur in infants, children and adults as well. Sepsis diagnosed in children less than 1 month old is specified by the term "Sepsis of Newborn".

Definition

Neonatal sepsis is a clinical syndrome which represents a general reaction to infection. It is characterized by systemic inflammation and general damage of tissues. Clinical definition is based on existing infection and systemic inflammatory response. Neonatal sepsis is diagnosed on the bases of clinical or microbiological data. Neonatal sepsis is an irreversible process which may cause mortality in cases of untimely detection and treatment.

Which symptoms are specific for sepsis in newborns?

- Fever, though some children may have low or normal body temperature
- Breathing problems or fast heart rate
- Baby feeds poorly
- Vomiting
- Jaundice (baby's skin or white tunic of eyes turn a yellowish tinge)
- Somnolence (difficulty in waking the child)
- Fingers and lips remain cyanotic (blue or purple coloration in the skin)

Danger signs:

When is it necessary to contact the doctor?

You should contact your pediatrician if your baby has one of above-listed symptoms or looks sick.

Is there a need to conduct laboratory tests on a child?

Yes, the doctor will ask: About the symptoms the baby has, previous deliveries and the baby's status at birth. Observation of child will be conducted and blood analysis of the child will be done including tests known as 'Blood Inoculation'. These tests may determine the existence of infection in the blood.

Frequently, there is need to conduct further laboratory testing in order to determine the existence of infection in different parts of body. Examples of some of these tests may be:

Lumbar Puncture (During this procedure doctor inject a thin needle into the lower part of backbone to obtain a small amount of spinal fluid. Lumbar liquid helps diagnose disease in the brain and spinal cord), analysis of urine, X-ray of thorax.

What kind of treatment is conducted for newborns with sepsis?

Most treatment is conducted in hospitals. Doctor will prescribe antibiotics (drug against infection) for your baby. The drug is given intravenously via a tube called an 'IV'.

Algorithm of management for suspected neonatal sepsis

Note: 1 ml. is sufficient for bacterial analysis of blood if a pediatric bottle is used. All material will be used for aerobic culture therefore anaerobic organisms rarely cause early neonatal sepsis. If there is a catheter, blood is obtained simultaneously from the central and peripheral catheter.

It is desirable that diagnostic tests be repeated 24 hours after the first examination. [11]

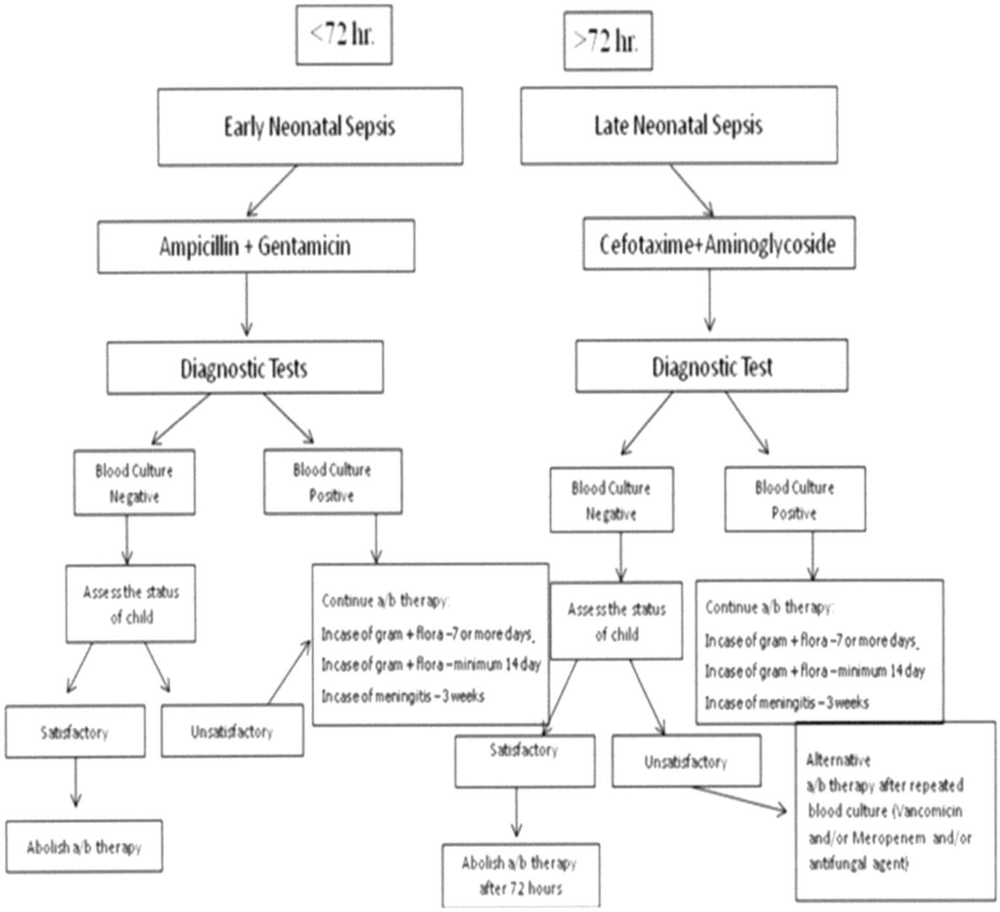

Figure 7. Therapeutic guidelines in neonatal infection 2011[11]

12. Conclusions and recommendations

1. Neonatal sepsis requires the immediate diagnosis and treatment in neonates regardless of gestational age or body weight at birth.
2. It is classified as early (<72hr) and late (>72hr); Late-late sepsis or Very Late Sepsis developing after 3 months of life in premature neonates with immune deficiencies.
3. Group B streptococcus (GBS) and staphylococcus are the most frequent agents of neonatal sepsis.
4. Risk factors of neonatal sepsis include GBS bacteriuria at ongoing pregnancy (>104 cfu/mL), colonization of mothers by GBS, duration of anhydrous interval ≥18 hours, mother's temperature at delivery ≥38º.
5. Non-specific and various clinical symptoms.
6. Evaluation of neonates if sepsis is suspected, must include perinatal anamnesis, full physical examination and laboratory tests including CBA with leukogram, blood culture, lumbar puncture for the exception of meningitis before a/b therapy starts,

culture of urine when the age of neonate is at least 6 days old and a culture obtained from other possible infections of nidus.

7. Differential diagnosis of sepsis must be conducted with other suspected systemic infections, neonatal hypoxia, congenital metabolic abnormalities of metabolism and neonatal respiratory distress.

Despites the fact that full-term and premature neonates acquiring sepsis is low, the possibility of serious consequences including death is so high that there is the need to conduct an immediate diagnoses and treatment of possible sepsis in neonates regardless of gestational age or body weight at birth.

Author details

Ketevan Nemsadze
Georgian National Academy of Sciences, Georgia

13. References

[1] Nemsadze K. *"Neonatology"*, 2010

[2] Micah Bhatti, Alison Chu, Joseph R. Hageman, Michael Schreiber and Kenneth Alexander: "Future Directions in the Evaluation and Management of Neonatal Sepsis"; *Neoreviews* 2012;13;e103 DOI: 10.1542/neo.13-2-e103 http://neoreviews.aappublications.org/content/13/2/e103

[3] Jennifer R. Verani, MD, Lesley McGee, PhD, Stephanie J. Schrag, DPhil: Centers for Disease Control and Prevention (CDC): *"Prevention of Perinatal Group B Streptococcal Disease RevisedGuidelines*(GBS)": http://www.cdc.gov/groupbstrep/guidelines/new-differences.html (2010)

[4] Hammad A. Ganatra, MBBSa, Barbara J. Stoll, MDb,Anita K.M. Zaidi, MBBS,*Sma "International Perspective on Early-Onset Neonatal Sepsis"*; 2010

[5] Stoll BJ, Hansen N, Fanaroff AA, et al. Late-onset sepsis in very low birth weight neonates: the experience of the NICHD neonatal research network. Pediatrics. 2002;110:285-291.

[6] J. Garcia-Prats et al., Semin*"Pediatric Infectional Disease"*, 20 00;11:4

[7] *Hotchsepsis. Department of Anestkiss RS, Karl IE, The pathophysiology and treatment of hesiology, Washington University School of Medicine, 2003*

[8] Sharma, S. & Mink, S. (2004). Emedicine: *"Septic Shock"*. http://www.emedicine.com/MED/topic2101.htm (Accessed February 14, 2006)

[9] Gabay C, Kushner I. *"Acute-phase proteins and other systemic responses to inflammation"*. New England Journal of Medicine; 1999;340(6):448–4; with permission

[10] Orr, P.A., Case, K.O., & Stevenson, J..J. *"Metabolic response and parenteral nutrition in trauma sepsis and burns Journal of Infusion Nursing"*; 2002. 25(1), 45-53. Retrieved March 7, 2006 from Ovid database

[11] *"Therapeutic guidelines in neonatal infection".2011*

[12] *J. Klein, S. Marcy. "Bacterial sepsis and meningitis". Mosby, 1995*

[13] William E. Benitz, MAdjunct." *Laboratory Tests in the Diagnosisof Early-OnsetNeonatal Sepsis";*2009

[14] *Neofax2009 Twenty Second Edition*

[15] Epidemiology and Diagnosis of Health Care-Associated Infections in the NICU, the Committee on Fetus and Newborn and the Committee on *Pediatrics* 2012;129;e1104 Infectious Diseases DOI: 10.1542/peds.2012-0147; http://pediatrics.aappublications.org/content/129/4/e1104.full.html

[16] Morven S Edwards, MD "Clinical features and diagnosis of sepsis in term and late preterm infants" updated: Dec 18, 2012 http://www.uptodate.com/contents/clinical-features-and-diagnosis-of-sepsis-in-term

Chapter 2

Neonatal Pneumonia

Friedrich Reiterer

Additional information is available at the end of the chapter

http://dx.doi.org/10.5772/54310

1. Introduction

Neonatal pneumonia is a serious respiratory infectious disease caused by a variety of microorganisms, mainly bacteria, with the potential of high mortality and morbidity (1,2). Worldwide neonatal pneumonia is estimated to account for up to 10% of childhood mortality, with the highest case fatality rates reported in developing countries (3,4). It´s impact may be increased in the case of early onset, prematurity or an underlying pulmonary condition like RDS, meconium aspiration or CLD/bronchopulmonary dysplasia (BPD), when the pulmonary capacity is already limited. Ureaplasma pneumonia and ventilator-associated pneumonia (VAP) have also been associated with the development of BPD and poor pulmonary outcome (5,6,7). In this chapter we will review different aspects of neonatal pneumonia and will present case reports from our level III neonatal unit in Graz.

2. Epidemiology

Reported frequencies of neonatal pneumonia range from 1 to 35 %, the most commonly quoted figures being 1 percent for term infants and 10 percent for preterm infants (8). The incidence varies according to gestational age, intubation status, diagnostic criteria or case definition, the level and standard of neonatal care, race and socioeconomic status. In a retrospective analysis of a cohort of almost 6000 neonates admitted to our NICU pneumonia was diagnosed in all gestational age classes. The incidence of bacterial pneumonia including Ureaplasma urealyticum (Uu) pneumonia was 1,4 % with a median patient gestational age of 35 weeks (range 23-42 weeks) and a mortality of 2,5%. There was only one case of viral pneumonia, due to RSV-infection and no case of fungal pneumonia. The mortality rate associated with pneumonia is in general inversely related to gestational age and birthweight, being higher in cases of early onset compared to late onset, and especially high in low socioecomomic groups and developing countries (2,3,4). Group B Streptococcus accounts for most cases of early onset pneumonia, the commonest bacteria causing late-onset pneumonia are gram-negative bacilli such as E coli or Klebsiella spp.(8). Frequently bacterial pathogens found in early and late onset sepsis/pneumonia are listed in Table 1.

3. Pathogenesis

Pneumonia may be acquired by intrauterine (e.g. transplacental hematogenous, ascending from birth canal), intrapartum (e.g aspiration) or postnatal routes (e.g. hematogenous, environmental). The pathogens include mainly bacteria, followed by viruses and fungi which induce an inflammatory pulmonary condition (1,8). This may cause epithelial injury to the airways, leakage of proteinaceous fluid into the alveoli and interstitium, leading to surfactant deficiency or dysfunction. Data from a German study (9) suggest that respiratory insufficiency in pneumonia is most likely caused by inhibition of surface-tension-lowering properties of surfactant rather than by surfactant deficiency. Important predisposing factors in the evolution of pneumonia are immaturity, low birth weight, premature rupture of membranes, chorioamnionitis and factors associated with prolonged neonatal intensive care (2, 8).

4. Clinical presentation, classification

Depending on the time of manifestation of infection neonatal pneumonia may be classified as early onset pneumonia (within the first 3 or 7 days of life, mostly within 48 hours), or late onset pneumonia (within 4 and 28 days of life). Congenital or intrauterine pneumonia can be considered a variant of early onset pneumonia (2). Other classifications refer to the underlying pathogen, like bacterial or viral pneumonia or the pattern of lung infiltrates (e.g. interstitial pneumonia) on chest radiographs. Clinical signs are unspecific and present as respiratory distress of various degree, suspicious appearing tracheal aspirates, cough, apnea, high or low temperature, poor feeding, abdominal distension, and lethargy. Tachypnea is a predominant clinical sign, present in 60-89 % of cases (2). Persistent fever is rather unusual, but has been reported in neonates with viral pneumonia (10). The radiographical appearance may also vary (11), showing reticulogranular-nodular infiltrates, and bilateral streaky or hazy lungs. As small bronchioli tend to collapse there may be compensatory hyperaeration in areas free of pneumonial infiltration. In addition there may be pleural effusions and/or pneumatocele formation in more complicated cases. Alveolar patterns with coarse, patchy parenchymal infiltrates, consolidation, and diffuse granularity are more typical for bacterial infections while parahilar streakiness, diffuse hazy lungs or reticulo-nodularity are more common in viral disease. The differential diagnoses to be considered on initial presentation are mainly surfactant deficiency syndrome and transient tachypnoe of the newborn, in addition meconium aspiration syndrome (MAS), pulmonary hemorrhage, pulmonary edema, primary pulmonary lymphangiectasis or pulmonary lymphangiomatosis, congestive heart failure (11,12) and Wilson-Mikity-syndrome (13). Additional investigations like echocardiography, high-resolution computed tomography, further laboratory studies, and in rare cases lung biopsy are helpful in the diagnostic work up.

5. Diagnosis

The clinical diagnosis of pneumonia is challenging and may not always be correct (over- or underestimated). Early tracheal aspirate cultures obtained within the first 8 to 12 hours of age may help in diagnosing congenital pneumonia (14,15), especially in certain clinical conditions, including maternal fever, clinical chorioamnionitis and leukopenia. But even a positive blood culture or proven airway colonization do not necessarily correlate with the clinical picture of sepsis or pneumonia (16). In the clinical routine pneumonia is diagnosed based on a combination of perinatal risk factors, signs of neonatal respiratory distress, positive laboratory studies, radiological signs and a typical clinical course. Some clinical scenarios are more or less suspicious . For example VAP, reported to be responsible for up to one third of all nosocomial infections, may be suspected two or more days after the initiation of mechanical ventilation when new or persistent infiltrates are noticed in 2 or more chest radiographs (5). Additional definition criteria developed by the Centers for disease control and prevention (17) include an increase in oxygen and ventilator requirements and at least three of the following signs and symptoms: temperature instability, wheezing, tachypnea, cough, abnormal heart rate, change in respiratory secretions, and abnormal peripheral white blood count. The most common organisms in VAP in extremely preterm infants have been shown to be Staphylococcus aureus and especially gram-negative organisms like Pseudomonas aeruginosa , Enterobacter spp. and Klebsiella spp. (18). Pneumonia caused by Ureaplasma species, Eubacteria mainly colonizing the mucosal surface of the respiratory and urogenital tract, may be diagnosed by direct isolation of the organism from endotracheal aspirates using culture or PCR-techniques, by typical chest-x-ray patterns showing disseminated, patchy infiltrates bilaterally with progression to cystic dysplasia, and elevated inflammatory serum-parameters like CRP or an increased white cell count (19,20,21). An organism frequently associated with early onset pneumonia is Group B Streptococcus. The clinical manifestation occurs usually within 6 of 8 hours of life and can initially mimic surfactant deficiency syndrome (16, 22).

6. Treatment, prevention

As pneumonia is often associated with or non distinguishable from bacterial sepsis initial therapy at the NICU includes broad spectrum intravenous antibiotics according to local protocols. In our unit we start with a combination of ampicillin and a second generation cephalosporine. Although there is no evidence from randomized controlled trials that any antibiotic regime is superior for suspected early onset neonatal sepsis (23), the WHO recommends as first line treatment ampicillin plus gentamycin (24). In cases where we detect pathogens in blood, or in endotracheal aspirates we treat according to susceptibility from antibiogram results. A problem which is increasing worldwide in NICU's is the occurrence of multidrug resistant pathogens, mainly gram-negative bacilli (25). As an alternative to systemic treatment aerosolized antibiotics like colistin have been used successfully in patients with VAP caused by multidrug resistant gram negative bacteria (26, 27). In patients where we suspect or diagnose an U infection we initiate treatment with intravenous clarithromycin (10mg/kg/day), a macrolid antibiotic. In a recently published randomized controlled placebo single-center study clarithromycin treatment resulted in eradication of Uu in 68,5 % of the patients and a significantly lower incidence of BPD (2.9% vs. 36.4%) in preterm infants weighing between 750 to 1250 g (28). Azithromycin, another macrolid antibiotic, which has good inhibitory activity against Ureaplasma in in-vitro studies, may also be beneficial for BPD prevention in Ureaplasma colonized/infected preterm infants, especially when used early and for longer duration (29). In general the clinical and microbiological effectiveness of macrolid antibiotics, the most commonly used in the literature being erythromycin, has not yet been shown in adequately powered randomized controlled clinical trials (30). Recommendations for the duration of antibiotic therapy in proven neonatal pneumonia range from 10 to 21 days (8). Surfactant therapy may be beneficial in selected patients by mechanisms improving lung function and decreasing bacterial growth, but may require repeated doses (22, 31,32). However, in a recently published meta- analysis in patients > 35 weeks gestation with proven or suspected pneumonia with onset during the first 28 days of life there was no evidence of a significant effect on the primary outcome death, time to resolution of pneumonia, BPD, pneumothorax and pulmonary hemorrhage (33). There are still open questions related to the surfactant preparation, dosage, optimal treatment frequency, number of doses and patient selection. Severe cases of pneumonia with respiratory insufficiency not responding to conventional therapy may occasionally be candidates for ECMO (34, 35). Preventative measures to be considered include maternal infection control in the prenatal period, prenatal screening and prophylaxis for streptococcal colonization (36), preference of non-or minimal invasive procedures in the neonatal period like respiratory support without intubation (37), immunoprophylaxis against RSV-infection, and general infection control measures in the neonatal unit to reduce the incidence and transmission of health-care-associated infections, the most important being hand hygiene (38,39,40). Preventive strategies that may have a great impact are maternal and infant vaccination programs, as has been already shown in developing countries e.g for pneumococcal polysaccharide vaccines (41).

Early onset (< =7 days)	Late onset (> 7 days)
Group B Streptococcus (g +)	Escherichia coli (g-)
Escherichea coli (g-)	Staphylococcus epidermidis (g+)
Staphylococcus aureus (g+)	Klebsiella-Enterobacter-species (g-)
Listeria monocytogenes (g+)	Pseudomonas aeruginosa (g-)
Enterococcus (g +)	
Ureaplasma urealyticum (g+)*	

g +/- = gram-positive/negative
* based on DNA-analysis

Table 1. Frequently found bacterial organisms in early and late onset neonatal sepsis and pneumonia

Case 1

A male neonate was born at 42 weeks gestational age to a multiparous healthy mother following spontaneous labor in an external hospital. The membranes ruptured 3 hours before delivery. There was no prenatal maternal screening for groub B streptococci disease.

After good primary transition, the infant developed clinical signs of respiratory distress with oxygen dependency and respiratory acidosis (6 hours post partum). After initiation of our standard broad spectrum antibiotic therapy the infant was transferred to our NICU. A septic workup showed leukopenia of 2.70 G/L, a left shift in the white cell count (immature/total neutrophils (I/T) 0,33), markedly elevated procalcitonin (303 ng/mL) and interleukin-6 (IL-6 > 400 pg/L) levels, but normal CRP values, and a positive urinary group B streptococcus testing. Blood cultures and tracheal aspirates were negative. Radiographics showed bilateral reticulogranular patterns compatible with the diagnosis of RDS (Figure 1). The patient was first placed on nasal CPAP but had to be intubated and ventilated mechanically due to respiratory deterioration with an increasing oxygen demand up to an FiO2 of 1,0 and persistent respiratory acidosis. Surfactant therapy showed no sufficient response. Inotropic support was necessary in case of arterial hypotension. Following inhaled nitric oxide therapy a decrease in oxygen requirement from 100 to 50 % was achieved over the following 48 hours, indicative of secondary pulmonary hypertension. On day 5 of life the clinical course was complicated by formation of a large left sided pneumatocele (Figure 2) and a consecutive symptomatic tension pneumothorax (Figure 3), which was successfully treated by insertion of a chest drain. On day 11 of life the patient was extubated, but the chest drain had to be left in situ for 3 ½ weeks due to recurrent air leaks. Laboratory parameters normalized within a week by our standard antibiotic regime. On day 37 of life the neonate had recovered and was discharged home.

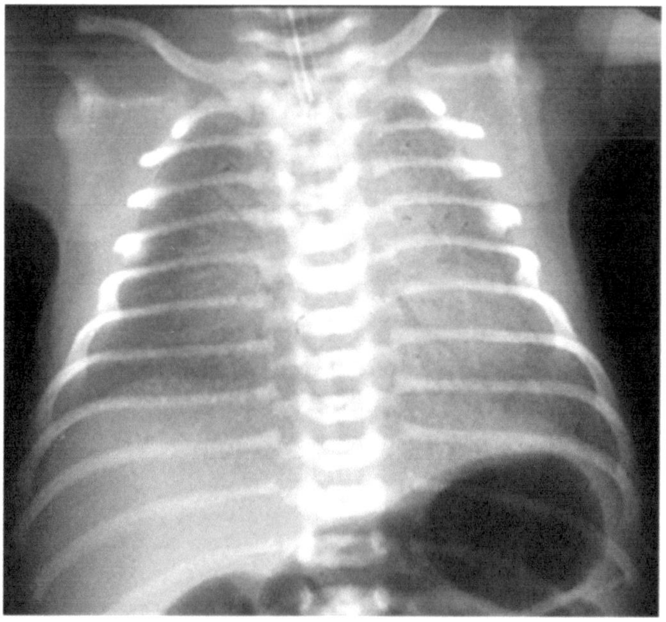

Figure 1. Bilateral reticulogranular lung pattern in Group B Streptococcus pneumonia mimicking RDS (Case 1)

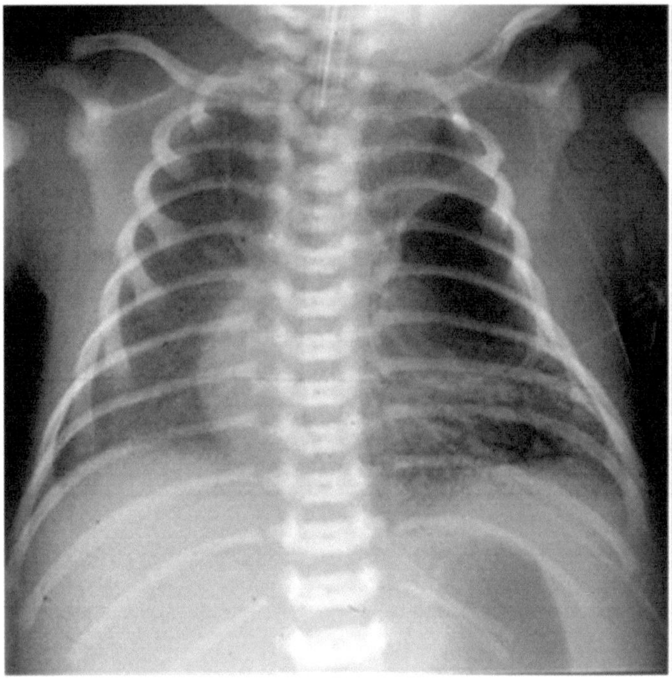

Figure 2. Pneumatocele formation on the leftside and streaky-granular infiltrates in Group B Streptococcus pneumonia (Case 1)

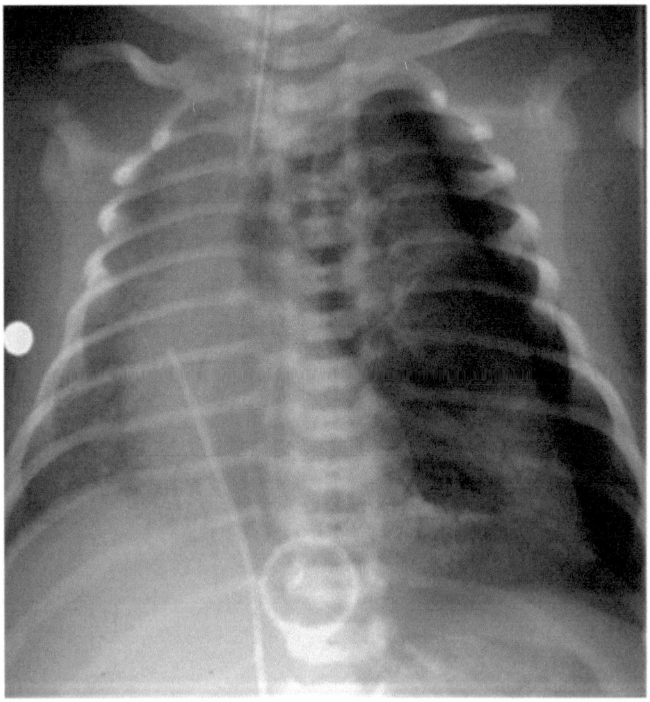

Figure 3. Leftsided tension pneumothorax complicating Group B Streptococcus pneumonia (Case 1)

Case 2

A female infant was delivered by vacuum extraction at 37+4 weeks gestational age to a multiparous mother after premature rupture of membranes, meconium stained amniotic fluid and pathological cardiotocogram. Maternal vaginal swabs were tested negative for Group B Streptococcus. Apgar scores and umbilical artery pH were within the normal range. About 12 hours after birth the neonate showed signs of respiratory distress with tachypnea, grunting and an oxygen demand of FiO2 >0,3. He was intubated and transferred to our NICU. A chest radiograph on admission showed bilateral streaky infiltrates (Figure 4). On day 2 an elevated CRP of 100mg/L, in combination with the findings on chest radiographs and the clinical signs were highly suspicious for the diagnosis of early onset neonatal pneumonia. In the yellowish tracheal aspirates Listeria monocytogenes were detected. The asymptomatic mother was tested negative for Listeria infection in stool and urine probes. On closer questioning the mother remembered having

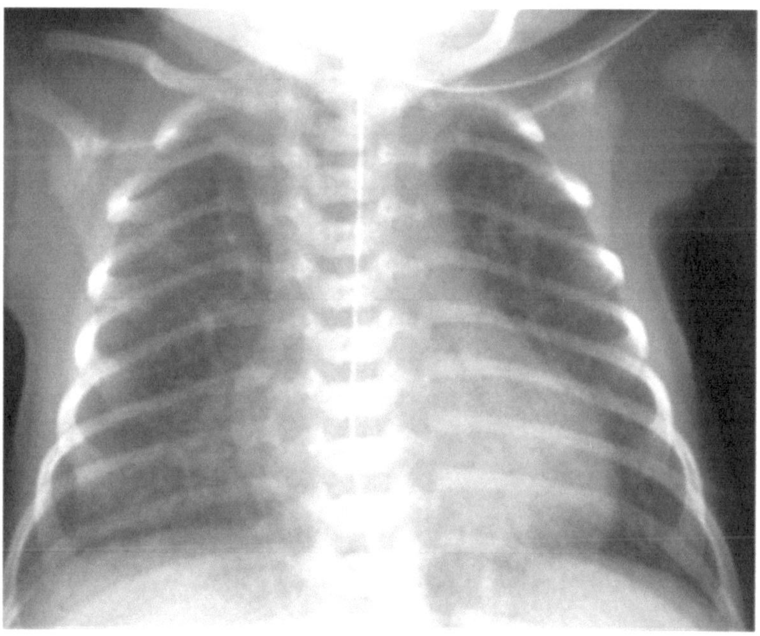

Figure 4. Bilateral,streaky and nodular infiltrates in Listeria pneumonia (Case 2)

developed gastrointestinal symptoms with diarrhea 2 weeks prior to birth after having eaten some cheese made from unpasteurized milk from a local food store. This led us to assume that the pregnant mother had most likely infected the fetus following ingestion of the bacterium, which had then crossed intestinal cells into the bloodstream and passed the placenta (42,43). After initiation of our standard antibiotic therapy the infant recovered quickly and was extubated on day 4 of life. Antibiotics were given for a total of 14 days. The child had a full recovery.

Case 3

A female infant was born to a primigravid mother at 28+1 weeks of gestational age. Delivery was by cesarean section due to a pathological cardiotocogram and presumed maternal infection (preterm premature rupture of the membranes 9 hours before delivery, preterm labour, increased neutrophile count and elevated CRP). The mother was treated with

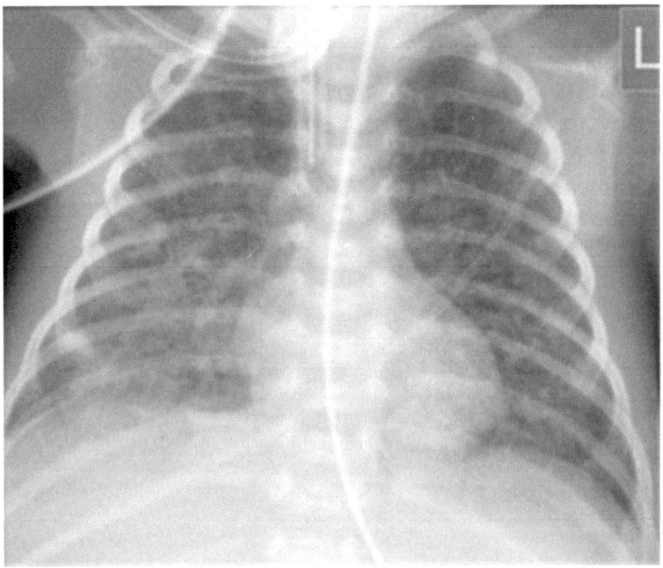

Figure 5. Bilateral lung infiltrates with consolidation mainly in the middle and right lower lobe in Enterobacter pneumonia (Case 3)

antibiotics. The preterm infant showed clinical and radiological signs of RDS and was intubated 15 minutes after birth. Standard broad spectrum antibiotics were started prophylactically but terminated after 3 days when daily white cell counts and CRP levels revealed no signs of infection. The patient was extubated on day 4 of life and placed on nasal CPAP. On day 6 of life the baby appeared septic with new onset of apneas, skin pallor, poor peripheral perfusion, metabolic acidosis and neurological signs like increased muscle tone and extreme irritability. Due to recurrent apneas despite caffeine therapy the infant had to be reintubated. The septic work up confirmed the clinical diagnosis of sepsis. Enterobacter cloacae, ESBL positive, was found in the blood culture, liquor cerebrospinalis and tracheal aspirate. Peripheral blood count showed leukocytosis, I/T ratio of 0,54, thrombocytopenia of 38 G/l, and elevated CRP values of 68,4 rising to a maximum of > 200 mg/L. Chest radiographs revealed new parenchymal changes compatible with the diagnosis of late onset bacterial pneumonia (Figure 5). The antibiotic regime was changed to meropenem and teicoplanin. As a further complication of sepsis the patient developed transient renal failure and an intraventricular hemorrhage with consecutive hydrocephalus, which was finally treated by insertion of a ventriculo-peritoneal shunt. After a long complicated neonatal period the patient was finally discharged from the hospital at an age of about 3 months in good clinical condition.

Case 4

A female infant was born at 24+3 weeks gestational age by vaginal delivery after the mother had been admitted to our hospital 1 hour prior to delivery with abdominal pain and onset of labors. The neonate developed RDS soon after birth which led to intubation, surfactant application and mechanical ventilation. Broad spectrum antibiotic therapy was started in case of suspected early onset sepsis. Initial laboratory revealed leukocytosis of 52.00 G/L, increased IL-6 (29,2 pg/ml) but normal CRP values. The chest radiograph on admission was typical for mild RDS but the lung pattern worsened during the first 2 weeks of life showing disseminated streaky-patchy infiltrates and partly cystic changes (Figure 6 and 7), accompanied by an increase in ventilatory requirements suggestive of early BPD changes. Therefore a strategy of moderate early BPD-prevention (48) with a one week course of intravenous steroids (hydrocortisone) was started. Results from routine tracheal aspirate screening for Ureaplasma infection taken during the second day on mechanical ventilation revealed a positive culture test (10^6) for Uu. In addition the placenta histology showed signs of chorioamnionitis. Under the assumption of early onset ureaplasma pneumonia/ pneumonitis we commenced oral macrolid therapy with clarithromycin (10mg/kg), beginning on day 6 of life for a total of 14 days. A repeat ureaplasma culture taken during treatment was negative. Mechanical ventilation continued for 18 days followed by a prolonged period of NCPAP lasting 7 weeks. Oxygen dependency for more than 8 weeks but not at a corrected gestational age of 36 weeks was compatible with the diagnosis of mild BPD (44,45). At an age of about 4 months of life she was discharged home.

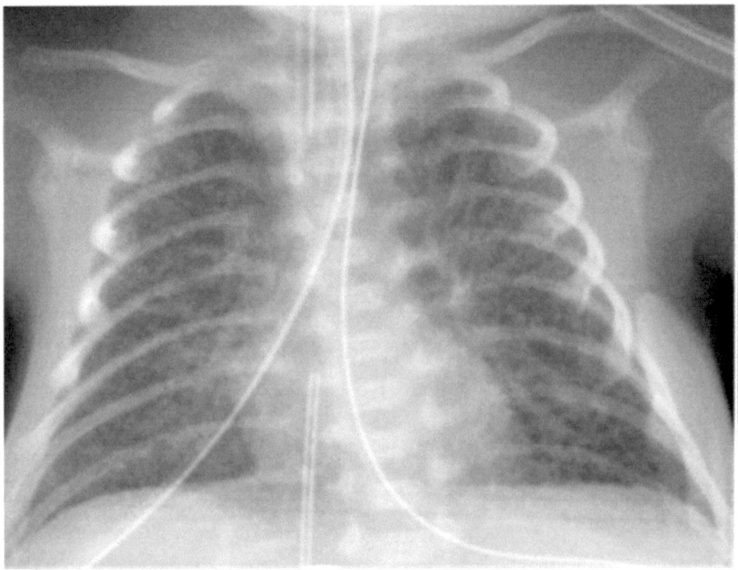

Figure 6. Streaky-patchy lung changes with partly cystic appearance in Ureaplasma urealyticum pneumonia on day 6 of life (Case 4)

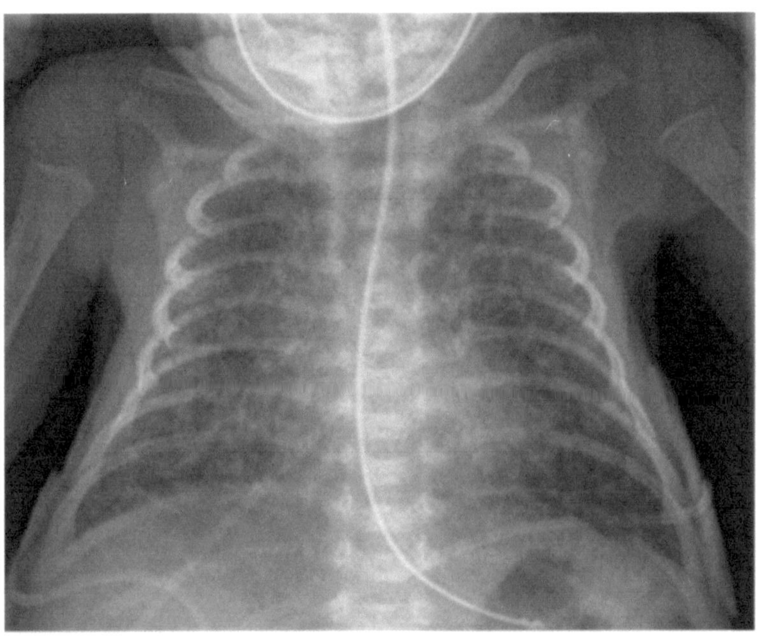

Figure 7. Early BPD changes in Ureaplasma urealyticum pneumonia on day 18 of life (Case 4)

7. Conclusion

Despite advances in neonatal medicine pneumonia remains a serious problem even in developed countries, mainly due to the increased survival of very preterm births and their susceptibility for early and late bacterial infections. The clinical spectrum of pneumonia is complex, symptoms are often non-specific and laboratory findings may be of limited value, making a rapid and correct diagnosis difficult. Treatment may also be challenging if no organism can be cultivated or in case of multidrug-resistant bacterial pneumonia. There is no clear evidence from randomized controlled trials favoring a specific antibiotic treatment strategy so that treatment decisions are based on local antimicrobial resistance patterns and clinical experience. Surfactant substitution might be beneficial in selected cases. Preventive strategies like health-care associated infection control and vaccination programs might have the greatest impact and should be further evaluated and applied at all levels of perinatal care.

Author details

Friedrich Reiterer
Division of Neonatology, Department of Pediatrics, Medical University of Graz, Austria

8. References

[1] Barnett ED, Klein JO. Bacterial infections of the respiratory tract. In: Remington JS, Klein JO (eds). Infectious diseases of the fetus and newborn infant. Philadelphia: WB Saunders, 5th edition 2001: 1006-1018.

[2] Nissen MD. Congenital and neonatal pneumonia. Pediatrics Resp. Reviews 2007; 8:195-203

[3] Duke T. Neonatal pneumonia in developing countries. Arch Dis Child Fetal Neonatal Ed.2005; 90: F2011-F219

[4] Black RE, Cousens S, Johnson HL et al. Global, regional, and national causes of child mortality in 2008: a systematic analysis, Lancet 2010; 375:1969-87

[5] RM Viscardi. Prenatal and postnatal microbial colonisation and respiratory outcome in preterm infants. In Bancalari E, Polin R. (eds). The newborn lung. 2nd edition, 2012; 6: 135-162

[6] Zhang HZ, Fang J, Su H et al. Risk factors for bronchopulmonary dysplasia in neonates born at < 1500g (1999-2009). Pediatrics International 2011; 53: 915-920

[7] Kotecha S, Hodge R, Schaber J et al. Pulmonary ureaplasma urealyticum is associated with the development of acute lung inflammation and chronic lung disease in preterm infants. Pediatr Res 2993; 61-68

[8] Dear PRF, FIFE A. Pneumonia. In: Greenough A, Milner AD.(eds). Neonatal respiratory disorders 2003; London: Arnold: 21: 278-310.

[9] Rüdinger M, Friedrich W, Rüstow B et al. Disturbed surfactant properties in preterm infants with pneumonia. Biol Neonate 2011;79:73-78

[10] Sert A, Yazar A, Odabas D et al. An unusual cause of fever in a neonate: Influenza A (H1N1) virus pneumonia. Pediatr Pulmonol 2010; 45:734-736.

[11] Swischuk LE. Imaging of the newborn, infant and young child. 3rd edition. Baltimore: William and Wilkins, 1989: 59-65

[12] Costa S, Rocha G, Leito A, Guimaraes H. Transient tachypnea of the newborn and congenital pneumonia: a comparative study. Journal of Maternal-Fetal and Neonatal Medicine 2012; 25; 7; 992-994

[13] Reiterer F, Dornbusch HJ, Urlesberger B et al. Cytomegalovirus associated neonatal pneumonia and Wilson-Mikity-syndrome: a causal relationship ?. Eur Resp. J 1999; 13: 460-462

[14] Booth GR, Al-Hosni M, Ali A et al. The utility of tracheal aspirate cultures in the immediate neonatal period. J Perinatal 2009; 29(7): 493-496

[15] Sherman MP, Goetzman BW, Ahlfors ChE. Tracheal aspirates and its clinical correlates in the diagnosis of congenital pneumonia. Pediatrics 1980: 65:2:258-263

[16] Webber S, Wilkinson AR, Lindsell D et al. Neonatal pneumonia, Arch Dis Child 1990;65:207-211

[17] Centers for Disease Control and Prevention. Criteria for defining nosocomial pneumonia. Available at:
htpp:// www.cdc.go/ncidodo/hip/NNIS/members/pneumonia/final/Pneu

[18] Apisarnthanarek A, Holsmannn-Pazgal G, Hamvas A et al. Ventilator associated pneumonia in extremely preterm neonates in an neonatal intensive care unit: characteristics, risk factors, and outcomes. Pediatrics. 2003; 112:1283-1289

[19] Waites KB, Schelonka RL,Xiao L et al. Congenital and opportunistic infections: Ureaplasma species and mycoplasma hominis. Seminars in Fetal & Neonatal Medicine 2009; 14:190-199

[20] Zotter H, Urlesberger B, Reiterer F et al. Ureaplasmapneumonien und Nachweis von ureaplasma urealyticum im Tubussekret bei Früh-und Neugeborenen. Gynäkol Geburtshilfliche Rundsch 1999; 39:191-194

[21] Moriokoa I, Fujibayashi H.Enoki E et al. Congenital pneumonia with sepsis caused by intrauterine infection of ureaplasma parvum in a term newborn: a first case report. J Perinatol.2010; 30 (5): 359-362

[22] Speer Ch, Sweet D. Surfactant Replacement: present and future. In Bancalari E, Polin R. (eds). The newborn lung. Neonatology questions and controversies. 2nd edition 2012; 14: 283-299.

[23] Mtitimila EI, Cooke RW. Antibiotic regimes for suspected early neonatal sepsis. The Cochrane library 2004; Issue 4.

[24] World Health Organization. Management of the child with a serious infection or severe malnutrition: Guidelines for care at first referral level in developing countries. Geneva: WHO, 2000.

[25] Patel SJ, Saiman L. Antibiotic resistance in neonatal intensive care unit pathogens: mechanism, clinical impact, and prevention including antibiotic stewardship. Clin Perinatol 2010; 37: 547-563

[26] IH Celik H, Oguz SS, Demirel G et al. Outcome of ventilator-associated pneumonia due to multidrug-resistant Acinetobacter baumannii and Pseudomonas aeruginosa treated with aerosolized colistin in neonates: a retrospective study. Eur J Pediatr 2012; 171:311-316
[27] Nakwan N, Wannaro J, Thongmak T et al. Safety in treatment of ventilator-associated pneumonia due to extensive drug-resistant acinetobacter baumannii with aerosolized colistin in neonates: A preliminary report. Pediatr Pulmonol 2011; 46: 60-66
[28] Ozdemir R, Erdeve O, Dizdar EA et a. Clarithromycin in preventing bronchopulmonary dysplasia in ureaplasma urealyticum-positive preterm infants. Pediatrics 2011; 128: e1496-e1501
[29] Ballard HO, Shook LA, Bernard P et al. Use of azithromycin for the prevention of bronchopulmonary dysplasia in preterm infants. Pediatr Pulmonol.2011; 46: 111-118
[30] Mabanta CG, Pryhuber GS, Weinberg GA at al. Erythromycin for the prevention of chronic lung disease in intubated preterm infants at risk for, or colonized with uraplasma urealyticum. Cochrane Database Syst Rev.2003; 4(4): CD003744
[31] Herting E, Gefeller O, Land M, et al. Surfactant treatment of neonates with respiratory failure and group B streptococcal infection. Members of the Collaborative European Multicenter-Study Group. Pediatrics 2000; 106:957-964.
[32] Finer NN. Surfactant use for neonatal lung injury: beyond respiratory distress syndrome. Paediatr Resp.Rev.2004; 5: Suppl A: S289-97
[33] Tan K, Lai NM, Sharma A. Surfactant for bacterial pneumonia in late preterm and term infants. Cochrane Database of Systematic Reviews. 2012, Issue 2, Art.No.CD008155
[34] Reiterer F, Kuttnig-Haim M, Maurer U et al. Erfolgreiche Behandlung einer therapierefraktären Schocklunge bei einem Neugeborenen mit connatalen Varicellen mittels Extracorporealer Membranoxygenierung. Klin Pädiatrie 1994; 206; 92-94.
[35] Malhotra A, Hunt R.W, Doherty R.R. Streptococcus pneumoniae sepsis in the newborn. Journal of Paediatrics Child Health 2010; 48: E79-E83
[36] Verani JR, Schrag SJ. Group B streptococcal disease in infants: progression in prevention and continued challenges. Clin Perinatol 2010; 37:375-392
[37] Garland JS. Strategies to prevent ventilator-associated pneumonia in neonates. Clinics in Perinatology 2010: 37: 629-643
[38] Abadesso C, Almeida HI, Virella D et al. Use of palizumab to control an outbreak of syncytial respiratory virus in a neonatal intensive care unit. J Hosp Infect 2004; 58(1):38-1
[39] Graham PL. Simple strategies to reduce health care associated infections in the neonatal unit: line, tube, and hand hygiene. Clinics in Perinatology 2010: 37: 645-653
[40] Kanmaz G, Erdeve O, Oguz SS et al. Influenza A (H1N1) virus pneumonia in newborns: experience of a referral level III neonatal intensive care unit in turkey. Pediatric Pulmonol 2011; 46: 201-202
[41] O`Dempsey BP, McArdle T, Ceesay SJ et al. Immunization with pneumococcal polysaccharides vaccine during pregnancy. Vaccine 1996; 14: 963-970
[42] Jasser-Nitsche H, Reiterer F, Kutschera J et al. Listerienpneumonie bei einem reifen Neugeborenen. Monatszeitschr Kinderheilkunde 2009; Suppl 2: 217-218

[43] Posfay-Barbe KM, Eald E. Listeriosis. Seminars in Fetal & Neonatal Medicine 2009; 14: 228-223

[44] Kugelman A, Durand M. A comprehensive approach to the prevention of brochopulmonary dysplasia. Pediatr Pulm 2011; 1-13

[45] Kinsella JP, Greenough A, Abmann SH. Bronchopulmonary dysplasia. Lancet 2006; 367: 1421-1431.

Chapter 3

Neonatal Osteomyelitis

Ursula Kiechl-Kohlendorfer and Elke Griesmaier

Additional information is available at the end of the chapter

http://dx.doi.org/10.5772/54320

1. Introduction

Acute osteomyelitis, although a rare complication in neonates, is a diagnostic and therapeutic challenge. Due to their immature immune response neonates are more susceptible to osteomyelitis than are older children. Preterm infants are at high risk for osteomyelitis because of frequent blood drawing, invasive monitoring/procedures and intravenous drug administration [1,2]. Early diagnosis of neonatal osteomyelitis might be difficult because of the paucity of clinical signs and symptoms, but has to be included in the differential diagnosis when late-onset or prolonged neonatal sepsis is present, as outcome is dependent on rapid diagnosis and immediate start of treatment.

2. Epidemiology

In Western countries the incidence of osteomyelitis and septic arthritis is 5-12 per 100.000 infants [3]. The overall incidence rate for bone and joint infections is 0.12 per 1000 live births and 0.67 per 1000 neonatal intensive care (NICU) admissions [4], with a mortality rate of 7.3% [5]. Some recent studies have reported an estimated incidence of 1-7 per 1000 hospital admissions for neonatal osteomyelitis [6,7]. In a review of more than 300 cases of neonatal osteomyelitis male infants are seen to predominate over females (1.6:1) and preterm infants to be at higher risk than term infants [8-10]. Risk factors for osteomyelitis and septic arthritis in preterm infants are mostly iatrogenic, including invasive procedures, intravenous or intra-arterial catheters, parenteral nutrition, ventilatory support, and bacteremia with nosocomial pathogens [11,12]. Two subgroups of neonates are affected: premature neonates with prolonged hospitalization and otherwise healthy newborns presenting within 2 to 4 weeks of discharge [13].

3. Microbiology

Neonatal osteomyelitis arises as a consequence of hematogenous spread of microorganisms, which is the most common route of infection. In preterm infants, neonatal osteomyelitis frequently results from directly inoculated bacteria (secondary to heel or venipuncture, umbilical catheterization, infected cephalhematoma, etc.) [14,15]. Premature rupture of membranes and transplacental infection have also been described as risk factors for neonatal osteomyelitis [16].

The most common bacterial pathogen causing osteomyelitis in children is *Staphylococcus aureus* in all age groups [17]. Group B streptococcus (Streptococcus agalactiae) and gram-negative organisms (E. coli and Klebsiella pneumonia) are also important bacteria in the neonatal period [16,18,19]. Community-acquired strains of methicillin-resistant *Staphylococcus aureus* have emerged as being relevant in recent years and cause serious infections in the neonate [12,20,21].

4. Pathogenesis

Hematogenous infection of the long bones, which are most frequently affected, begins in the capillary loops of the metaphysic, adjacent to the cartilaginous growth plate (physis). These areas are very susceptible to hematogenous infection, because of its high vascularity and because the blood flow within the vessels is slow [22]. Bacteria can pass through gaps from the sinusoidal veins to the capillaries into the tissue, where they are provided an ideal environment to grow, resulting in abscess formation. These abscesses frequently rupture into the joint [23]. In neonates acute hematogenous osteomyelitis and septic arthritis co-exist in up to 76% of all cases as a result of this unique vascular anatomy of the epiphysis; the bone marrow compartment is seldom involved [10,24]. The epiphysis receives its blood supply directly from metaphyseal blood vessels (transphyseal vessels) and the adjacent cartilaginous growth plate is traversed by capillaries, allowing spread of the pathogenic bacteria to the physis, epiphysis and joint and resulting in slipped epiphyses, fractures, premature physeal closure and chronic infection (Figure 1) [25].

Characteristics of the neonatal bone prevent many of the features of chronic osteomyelitis: cortical sequestra are often completely absorbed due to extensive bone blood supply in the newborn and, in addition, efficient vasculature of the inner layer of the periosteum encourages early development of new bone formation [26,27]. Complete destruction of joints is rare, but serious growth disturbances may occur.

5. Diagnosis

Diagnosis of osteomyelitis in the neonate can be challenging and is often delayed, as it is rare in the neonatal period and frequently presents with non-specific signs of illness. Diagnosis is based on clinical signs and symptoms, laboratory findings, radiological and microbiological criteria.

5.1. Clinical signs and symptoms

In general, two distinct clinical syndromes have been postulated to be associated with neonatal osteomyelitis: 1) a benign form, with little or no evidence of infection other than local swelling, and 2) a severe form, with the predominant manifestation of a sepsis-like syndrome with multiple bone sites being noted as manifestations [28]. In neonates, almost half of all cases involve two or more bones.

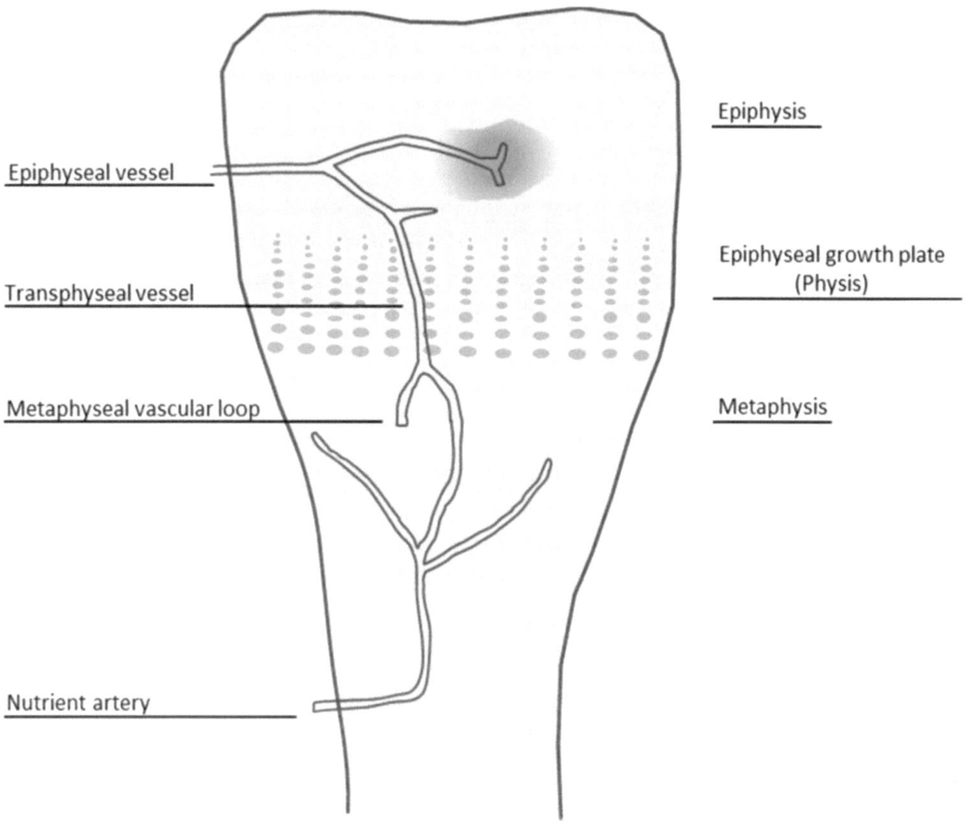

Figure 1. Anatomic depiction of blood supply to the epiphysis and metaphysis in the developing bone that influences the progression of osteomyelitis in the neonate (modified and redrawn from Kaye JJ et al, [53]).

Clinical symptoms and signs of osteomyelitis in the neonate are at first frequently unspecific and mild. They may include temperature instability, feeding intolerance, irritability or reduced movement, frequently giving rise to the suspicion of secondary sepsis. Fever is a rare condition that could be explained by a rather poorly developed immune system. As the disease progresses, more specific signs may become present, including disability, local swelling or erythema. Focal tenderness over a long bone should catch the physician's attention. In some cases subcutaneous abscess formation prompts the diagnosis of osteomyelitis. Hip, knee and shoulder are most frequently involved [7,28,29].

5.2. Laboratory findings

In general, there is no specific laboratory test for osteomyelitis. Neonates with osteomyelitis frequently show normal leukocyte counts and erythrocyte sedimentation rates in the first days. Thus, normal values do not preclude the diagnosis [30]. The C-reactive protein (CRP) is a rapid indicator of systemic inflammation and tissue damage, is useful as acute phase reactant, but not specific for skeletal infection. Procalcitonin has also been described as a potential marker in the diagnosis of osteomyelitis in children, but needs to be investigated in larger trials, especially in newborns [31,32]. Elevated values of CRP and erythrocyte sedimentation rates could be used to monitor response to therapy or identify complications.

5.3. Imaging techniques

Radiological investigations confirm the suspicion of neonatal osteomyelitis, define the infection site, differentiate between unifocal and multifocal disease patterns and identify secondary complications. Computed tomography, magnetic resonance imaging, ultrasound, radiography and bone scintigraphy scanning have been reported to be useful in detecting osteomyelitis. However, awareness of radiation exposure, need for sedation and transfer to another unit must be considered in the selection of technique.

Radiographs should be the first diagnostic assessment to be performed in patients with suspected osteomyelitis, because they may suggest the correct diagnosis and exclude other pathologic conditions (Figure 2a). However, the specificity of plain radiographs for detecting osteomyelitis is greater (75% to 83%) than its sensitivity (43% to 75%) [33]. Plain radiography can show soft tissue swelling and destroyed fascial planes within days after onset of infection, but may be subtle and not obvious until day 5 to 7 in children [34]. In the neonate even soft tissue swelling may not be present, because subcutaneous fat is lacking and fascial planes are poorly defined. Joint effusions might be suspected if widening of the joint space or bulging of the soft tissues is detected. Additional early changes are as follows: periosteal thickening/elevation, lytic lesions, osteopenia, loss of trabecular architecture, and new bone apposition [35]. Of importance, destructive bone changes do not appear until 7 to 14 days of disease [25].

Predominately in children, ultrasound can detect features of acute osteomyelitis several days earlier, than radiographs [34]. Even though findings may not be specific and standardized reports for neonates with osteomyelitis are lacking, ultrasound should be taken into account as a useful additional diagnostic tool for the early detection and management of osteomyelitis in neonates as it has many advantages: it is non-invasive, readily accessible, performed bedside, of minimal discomfort for the patient, does not use ionizing radiation and does not need sedation [36,37]. Even though ultrasound cannot exclude the diagnosis of osteomyelitis, its main value lies in its ability to identify involvement of the adjacent soft tissue (subperiosteal fluid collection or abscess formation), periosteal thickening or elevation, joint effusions and irregularities or interruptions of the cortical bone (Figure 2b) [38,39]. Color Doppler imaging further supports the diagnostic assessment, showing coexisting presence of hyperemia surrounding the periost and soft tissue abscess formation. Ultrasound can also be used to image guided-needle aspiration of the subperiosteal fluid for pathogenic organism isolation or subperiosteal abscess drainage. Furthermore, ultrasound has been described as being helpful in differentiating between epiphyseal separation and subluxation following septic arthritis [40]. However, ultrasound cannot exclude the diagnosis of acute osteomyelitis, and thus further imaging diagnostics may be required [41,42].

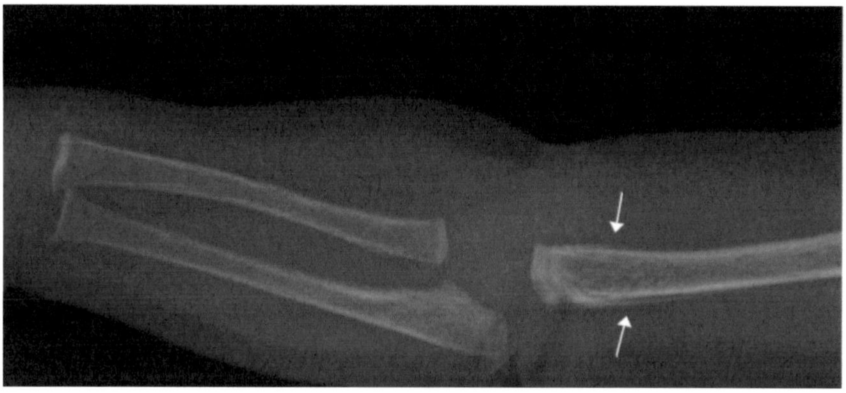

(a)

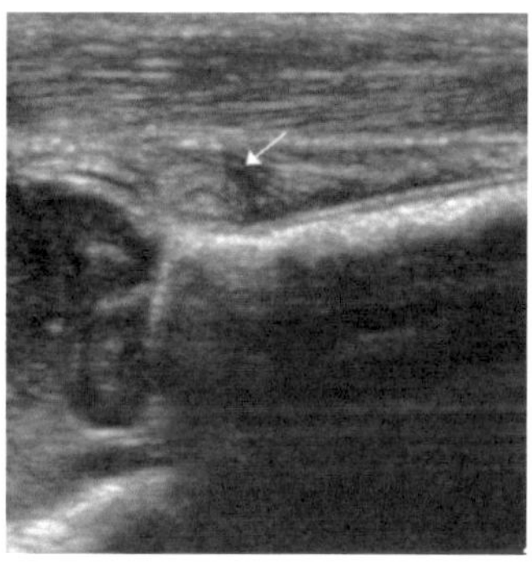

(b)

Figure 2. Acute osteomyelitis of the right humerus. **a)** periosteal elevation and soft tissue swelling **b)** joint effusion and synovial thickening

Magnetic resonance imaging (MRI) has high specificity (94%) and sensitivity (97%) for the diagnosis of acute osteomyelitis, showing changes as early as day 3 to 5 after the onset of infection [43,44]. MRI gives excellent tissue characterization and high resolution, showing detailed anatomic presence of the inflammatory process and its complications (abscess formation, physeal involvement, septic arthritis), further allowing the assessment of involvement of the growth plate and epiphysis. MRI has been proven useful in the diagnosis of clinically suspected osteomyelitis in children [45-48], but for its use in neonatology it has several limitations: first and foremost the need for sedation and transfer to the MRI unit.

Three-phase bone imaging, using technetium 99m is very sensitive (90%-95%) for the detection of acute osteomyelitis in the early stages of disease and allows detection within 24 to 48 hours after onset of symptoms [34,49]. Bone scintigraphy is especially useful for detecting multiple foci of infection or if the infection site is poorly localized. Technetium-99 methylene diphosphonate accumulates in areas of increased bone turnover and is for now the preferred agent of choice for radionuclide bone imaging. In neonates bone scintigraphy is the subject of controversy: only a few reports support its use and have shown that sensitivity is much lower, than in older infants because of poor bone mineralization [18,48,50].

6. Treatment

Successful cure of osteomyelitis during the newborn period is dependent on a fast and true diagnosis and sufficient treatment. Empirical selection of antibiotic therapy depends on the age and the clinical situation of the infant. Antimicrobial therapy should be started as soon as the diagnosis is made and directed against the most common bacterial isolates responsible for hematogenous osteomyelitis according to age group. Delay in therapy commencement increases the risk for complications. If a definitive organism is isolated, antimicrobial treatment should be accordingly adjusted.

For neonates an empiric regimen should include excellent coverage against S. aureus, group B streptococcus and enteric gram-negative bacteria, thus consisting of a third-generation cephalosporin (cefotaxime) plus an antistaphylococcal agent (amoxicillin). Infants at risk for hospital-acquired infection (methicillin-resistant or coagulase negative Staphylococcus aureus) should receive vancomycin instead of amoxicillin.

Duration of treatment depends on the extent of infection, the clinical response and the presence of underlying risk factors [51]. In the case of unifocal osteomyelitis continuation of treatment for six weeks and in the case of complex disease, defined as multifocal, significant bone destruction, resistant unusual pathogen, septic shock, continuation for more than six weeks to months might be required. Antimicrobial treatment is frequently administered intravenously for two to three weeks and then switched to oral medication [52]. Surgery is indicated to drain acute abscesses or when no improvement is achieved with antibiotic treatment.

7. Prognosis

Several studies have documented poor outcome even with modern treatment facilities. In neonates the reported incidence of permanent sequelae varies from 6% to 50% [2,11]. Neonatal osteomyelitis can lead to permanent joint disabilities, disturbances in bone growth secondary to damage to the cartilaginous growth plate, limb-length discrepancies, arthritis, decreased range of motion and pathologic fractures [51].

8. Conclusion

Neonatal osteomyelitis, although a rare complication, remains a diagnostic and therapeutic challenge and poses the infant at high risk for long term morbidity. Osteomyelitis should be considered in newborn infants presenting with clinical signs of sepsis, but lacking an obvious focus, in order to facilitate early diagnosis and prompt initiation of appropriate therapy.

Author details

Ursula Kiechl-Kohlendorfer and Elke Griesmaier
Department of Pediatrics II,
Medical University of Innsbruck,
Innsbruck, Austria

9. References

[1] Lim MO, Gresham EL, Franken EA Jr, Leake RD. Osteomyelitis as a complication of umbilical artery catheterization. Am J Dis Child. 1977;131(2):142-4.
[2] Williamson JB, Galasko CS, Robinson MJ. Outcome after acute osteomyelitis in preterm infants. Arch Dis Child. 1990;65:1060-2.
[3] Rasool MN. Hematogenous osteomyelitis of the calcaneus in children. J Pediatr Orthop. 2001;21(6):738-43.
[4] Ho NK, Low YP, See HF. Septic arthritis in the newborn--a 17 years' clinical experience. Singapore Med J. 1989;30(4):356-8.
[5] Caksen H, Oztürk MK, Uzüm K, Yüksel S, Ustünbaş HB, Per H. Septic arthritis in childhood. Pediatr Int. 2000;42(5):534-40.
[6] Goldmann DA, Durbin WA Jr, Freeman J. Nosocomial infections in a neonatal intensive care unit. J Infect Dis. 1981;144(5):449-59.
[7] Berberian G, Firpo V, Soto A, Lopez Mañan J, Torroija C, Castro G, Polanuer P, Espinola C, Piñeiro JL, Rosanova MT. Osteoarthritis in the neonate: risk factors and outcome. Braz J Infect Dis. 2010;14(4):413-8.
[8] De Boeck H. Osteomyelitis and septic arthritis in children. Acta Orthop Belg. 2005;71(5):505-15.
[9] Krogstad P. Osteomyelitis and septic arthritis. In: Feigin RD, Cherry JD, Demmler GJ, et al., eds. Textbook of Pediatric Infectious Diseases. Fifth edition. Philadelphia: Saunders 2004: 713–36.
[10] Fox L, Sprunt K. Neonatal osteomyelitis. Pediatrics. 1978;62(4):535-42.
[11] Frederiksen B, Christiansen P, Knudsen FU. Acute osteomyelitis and septic arthritis in the neonate, risk factors and outcome. Eur J Pediatr. 1993;152(7):577-80.
[12] Ish-Horowicz MR, McIntyre P, Nade S. Bone and joint infections caused by multiply resistant Staphylococcus aureus in a neonatal intensive care unit. Pediatr Infect Dis J. 1992;11(2):82-7.
[13] Dessì A, Crisafulli M, Accossu S, Setzu V, Fanos V. Osteo-articular infections in newborns: diagnosis and treatment. J Chemother. 2008;20(5):542-50.

[14] Bergdahl S, Ekengren K, Eriksson M. Neonatal hematogenous osteomyelitis: risk factors for long-term sequelae. J Pediatr Orthop. 1985;5(5):564-8.
[15] Wong M, Isaacs D, Howman-Giles R, Uren R. Clinical and diagnostic features of osteomyelitis occurring in the first three months of life. Pediatr Infect Dis J. 1995;14(12):1047-53.
[16] Liao SL, Lai SH, Lin TY, Chou YH, Hsu JF. Premature rupture of the membranes: a cause for neonatal osteomyelitis? Am J Perinatol. 2005;22(2):63-6.
[17] Asmar BI. Osteomyelitis in the neonate. Infect Dis Clin North Am. 1992;6(1):117-32.
[18] McPherson DM. Osteomyelitis in the neonate. Neonatal Netw. 2002;21(1):9-22.
[19] Qadir M, Ali SR, Lakhani M, Hashmi P, Amirali A. Klebsiella osteomyelitis of the right humerus involving the right shoulder joint in an infant. J Pak Med Assoc. 2010;60(9):769-71.
[20] Saavedra-Lozano J, Mejías A, Ahmad N, Peromingo E, Ardura MI, Guillen S, Syed A, Cavuoti D, Ramilo O. Changing trends in acute osteomyelitis in children: impact of methicillin-resistant Staphylococcus aureus infections. J Pediatr Orthop. 2008;28(5):569-75.
[21] Korakaki E, Aligizakis A, Manoura A, Hatzidaki E, Saitakis E, Anatoliotaki M, Velivasakis E, Maraki S, Giannakopoulou C. Methicillin-resistant Staphylococcus aureus osteomyelitis and septic arthritis in neonates: diagnosis and management. Jpn J Infect Dis. 2007;60(2-3):129-31.
[22] Green NE, Edwards K. Bone and joint infections in children. Orthop Clin North Am. 1987;18(4):555-76.
[23] Ogden JA, Light TR. Pediatric osteomyelitis: III. anaerobic microorganisms. Clin Orthop Relat Res. 1979;(145):230-6.
[24] Bergdahl S, Ekengren K, Eriksson M. Neonatal hematogenous osteomyelitis: risk factors for long-term sequelae. J Pediatr Orthop. 1985;5(5):564-8.
[25] Blickman JG, van Die CE, de Rooy JW. Current imaging concepts in pediatric osteomyelitis. Eur Radiol. 2004;14 Suppl 4:L55-64.
[26] Green WT, Shannon JG. Osteomyelitis of infants: a disease different from osteomyelitis of older children. Arch Surg. 1936;32:462.
[27] Trueta J. Three types of acute haematogenous osteomyelitis. J Bone Joint Surg Br. 1959;41:671.
[28] Overturf G, Marcy M. Bacterial infections of the bones and joints. In: Remington J and Klein J editors. Infectious diseases of the fetus and newborn infant, 5th edition 2001 WB Sounders. Chapter 23; 1019-103.
[29] Al Saadi MM, Al Zamil FA, Bokhary NA, Al Shamsan LA, Al Alola SA, Al Eissa YS. Acute septic arthritis in children. Pediatr Int. 2009;51(3):377-80.
[30] Mok PM, Reilly BJ, Ash JM. Osteomyelitis in the neonate. Clinical aspects and the role of radiography and scintigraphy in diagnosis and management. Radiology. 1982;145(3):677-82.

[31] Butbul-Aviel Y, Koren A, Halevy R, Sakran W Procalcitonin as a diagnostic aid in osteomyelitis and septic arthritis. Pediatr Emerg Care 2005;21(12):828-23.
[32] Faesch S, Cojocaru B, Hennequin C, Pannier S, Glorion C, Lacour B, Chéron G. Can procalcitonin measurement help the diagnosis of osteomyelitis and septic arthritis? A prospective trial. Ital J Pediatr. 2009;35(1):33.
[33] Christian S, Kraas J, Conway WF. Musculoskeletal infections. Semin Roentgenol. 2007;42(2):92-101.
[34] Pineda C, Espinosa R, Pena A. Radiographic imaging in osteomyelitis: the role of plain radiography, computed tomography, ultrasonography, magnetic resonance imaging, and scintigraphy. Semin Plast Surg. 2009;23(2):80-9.
[35] Kothari NA, Pelchovitz DJ, Meyer JS. Imaging of musculoskeletal infections. Radiol Clin North Am. 2001;39(4):653-71.
[36] Mah ET, LeQuesne GW, Gent RJ, Paterson DC.Ultrasonic features of acute osteomyelitis in children. J Bone Joint Surg Br. 1994;76(6):969-74.
[37] Howard CB, Einhorn M, Dagan R, Nyska M. Ultrasound in diagnosis and management of acute haematogenous osteomyelitis in children. J Bone Joint Surg Br. 1993;75(1):79-82.
[38] Abiri MM, Kirpekar M, Ablow RC. Osteomyelitis: detection with US. Radiology. 1989;172(2):509-11.
[39] Zawin JK, Hoffer FA, Rand FF, Teele RL. Joint effusion in children with an irritable hip: US diagnosis and aspiration. Radiology. 1993;187(2):459-63.
[40] Vasquez M. Osteomyelitis in children. Current Opinions in Pediatrics,2002;14: 112-5. 7
[41] Kleinman PK. A regional approach to osteomyelitis of the lower extremities in children. Radiol Clin North Am. 2002;40(5):1033-59.
[42] Pineda C, Vargas A, Rodríguez AV. Imaging of osteomyelitis: current concepts. Infect Dis Clin North Am. 2006;20(4):789-825.
[43] Mandell GA. Imaging in the diagnosis of musculoskeletal infections in children. Curr Probl Pediatr. 1996;26(7):218-37.
[44] Kocher MS, Lee B, Dolan M, Weinberg J, Shulman ST. Pediatric orthopedic infections: early detection and treatment. Pediatr Ann. 2006;35(2):112-22.
[45] Dangman BC, Hoffer FA, Rand FF, O'Rourke EJ. Osteomyelitis in children: gadolinium-enhanced MR imaging. Radiology. 1992;182(3):743-7.
[46] Mazur JM, Ross G, Cummings J, Hahn GA Jr, McCluskey WP.Usefulness of magnetic resonance imaging for the diagnosis of acute musculoskeletal infections in children. J Pediatr Orthop. 1995;15(2):144-7.
[47] Oudjhane K, Azouz EM. Imaging of osteomyelitis in children. Radiol Clin North Am. 2001;39(2):251-66.
[48] Jaramillo D, Treves ST, Kasser JR, Harper M, Sundel R, Laor T. Osteomyelitis and septic arthritis in children: appropriate use of imaging to guide treatment. AJR Am J Roentgenol. 1995;165(2):399-403.

[49] Ranson M. Imaging of pediatric musculoskeletal infection. Semin Musculoskelet Radiol. 2009;13(3):277-99.

[50] Guilbert J, Meau-Petit V, de Labriolle-Vaylet C, Vu-Thien H, Renolleau S. Coagulase-negative staphylococcal osteomyelitis in preterm infants: a proposal for a diagnostic procedure. Arch Pediatr. 2010;17(10):1473-6.

[51] Gutierrez K. Bone and joint infections in children. Pediatr Clin North Am. 2005;52(3):779-94.

[52] Faust SN, Clark J, Pallett A, Clarke NM. Managing bone and joint infection in children. Arch Dis Child. 2012 Jun;97(6):545-53.

[53] Kaye JJ, Winchester PH, Freiberger RH. Neonatal septic "dislocation" of the hip: true dislocation or pathological epiphyseal separation. Radiology 1975;114:671-674).

Section 2

Diagnostic Approaches

Chapter 4

The Role of C-Reactive Protein in the Diagnosis of Neonatal Sepsis

Nora Hofer, Wilhelm Müller and Bernhard Resch

Additional information is available at the end of the chapter

http://dx.doi.org/10.5772/54255

1. Introduction

During the last decades advances in neonatal intensive care have led to an impressive decrease of neonatal mortality and morbidity. However, infectious episodes in the early postnatal period still remain serious and potentially life-threatening events with a mortality rate of up to 50% in very premature infants. [1, 2] The signs and symptoms of neonatal sepsis can be clinically indistinguishable from various noninfectious conditions such as respiratory distress syndrome or maladaptation. Therefore rapid diagnosis is crucial for preventing the child from an adverse outcome. The current practice of starting empirical antibiotic therapy in all neonates showing infection-like symptoms results in their exposure to adverse drug effects, nosocomial complications, and in the emergence of resistant strains. [3]

Sepsis results from the complex interaction between the invading microorganism and the host immune, inflammatory, and coagulation response. [4, 5] Inflammatory cytokines (TNF-α, IL-1β, IL-6, IL-8, IL-15, IL-18, MIF) and growth factors (IL-3, CSFs), and their secondary mediators, including nitric oxide, thromboxanes, leukotrienes, platelet-activating factor, prostaglandins, and complement, cause activation of the coagulation cascade, the complement cascade, and the production of prostaglandins, leukotrienes, proteases and oxidants. [6]

Laboratory sepsis markers represent a helpful tool in the evaluation of a child with clinical signs and complement the evaluation of a neonate with a potential infection. During the last decades efforts were done to improve laboratory sepsis diagnosis and a variety of the above mentioned markers and more were studied with different success. Despite the promising results for some of them current evidence suggests that none of them can consistently diagnose 100% of infected cases. C-reactive protein (CRP) is the most extensively acute phase reactant studied so far and despite the ongoing rise (and fall) of new infection markers it still remains the preferred index in many neonatal intensive care units.

There is great interest in rapid diagnostic tests that are able to safely distinguish infected from uninfected newborns, especially in the early phase of the disease. [7] In fact, a delayed start of the antibiotic treatment may be no more able to stop the fulminant clinical course with development of septic shock and death within hours after the first clinical symptoms. [8] In the era of multi-resistant microorganisms, it is as well important to avoid the unnecessary use of antibiotics in sepsis-negative infants.

2. Structure and function of CRP

CRP was first described in 1930 by Tillet and Francis at Rockefeller University. [9] They observed a precipitation reaction between serum from patients suffering acute pneumococcal pneumonia and the extracted polysaccharide fraction C from the pneumococcal cell wall. This reaction could not be observed when using serum of neither healthy controls nor the same pneumonia patients after they had recovered. In view of the fact that the polysaccharide fraction was a protein the C-reactive component in the serum was named C-reactive protein. [9] By the 1950s CRP had been detected in more than 70 disorders including acute bacterial, viral, and other infections, as well as non-infectious diseases such as acute myocardial infarction, rheumatic disorders, and malignancies. [10] All of these disorders of disparate etiology had in common the theme of inflammation and/or tissue injury. [11]

CRP is composed by five identical subunits arranged in a cyclic pentameter shape. The whole protein has a diameter of 102 Å (1 Ångström = 10^{-10} m) and a molecular weight of 118 000 Daltons. [12] All subunits have the same orientation; therefore the whole protein has two faces, a 'recognition' face exhibiting five phosphocholin-binding sites and an 'effector' face containing complement and Fc-receptor-binding sites. [12] The principal ligand to CRP with the highest binding affinity is phosphocholin, which is found in lipopolysaccharid and cell walls of many bacteria and micro-organisms as well as in the outer leaflet of most biological membranes. [12]

After binding to a macromolecular ligand CRP is recognized by the component C1q of the complement system and activates it on the classical pathway. CRP-ligand complexes bind to the Fc-receptor on neutrophil granulocytes, macrophages, etc as well and thus promote phagocytosis of the pathogen. CRP further activates monocytes and macrophages and stimulates the production of pro-inflammatory cytokines such as Interleukin-1 and Tumor necrosis factor α. [12, 13]

3. CRP is part of the acute-phase-response

The acute-phase-response is a physiological and metabolic reaction to an acute tissue injury of different etiology (trauma, surgery, infection, acute inflammation, etc) which aims to neutralize the inflammatory agent and to promote the healing of the injured tissue. [11]

After a trauma or the invasion of microorganisms an acute localized inflammatory reaction is initiated by activation of local resident cells. The contact with bacterial endo-or exotoxins initiates the release of prostaglandins, leucotriens, and histamine, which results in vasodilatation, elevated vascular permeability, sensibilization of nozizeptors, and attraction and activation of further inflammatory cells.

Activated fibroblasts, leukocytes, and endothelial cells produce pro-inflammatory cytokines including IL-1, TNF- α, and IL-6. They are responsible for the development of fever, lethargy, arthralgia, and headache, they activate the vascular endothelial cells, regulate proliferation of T-and B-lymphocytes, activate macrophages, have pro-coagulatory effects on endothelial cells, and they induce the production of acute-phase-proteins in the hepatocytes of the liver.

Acute-phase-proteins form a heterogeneous group and include components of the complement system, coagulation factors, protease inhibitors, metal binding proteins, CRP, and other proteins that increase or decrease by more than 25% during an inflammatory reaction. [11-13]

The production of CRP in the hepatocytes is mainly induced by IL-6 but can be further increased by synergy with IL-1. [14]] Some authors have aimed to determine the normal serum CRP concentration in healthy adults: In 1981 Shine et al. [15] evaluated serum concentration of CRP determined by radioimmunoassay in 468 sera from normal adult volunteer blood donors and reported on a median concentration of 0.8 mg/l with a 90th percentile of less than 3.0 mg/l. More recently, Rifai and Ridker [16] used three different high-sensitivity techniques to determine CRP distributions in their cohort consisting of 22 thousand healthy adults from the Unites States. The median CRP values for men and women were 1.5 and 1.52 mg/l, the 90th percentiles were 6.05 and 6.61 mg/l, respectively. Similarly, Imhof et al [17] examined CRP values from 13 thousand apparently healthy men and women from different populations in Europe. The reported median concentration in the single cohorts ranged from 0.6 to 1.7 mg/l, the 90th percentiles from 3.2 to 8.0 mg/l.

During the acute-phase-response the hepatic synthesis rate increases within hours and can reach levels 1000 fold. [10, 12] CRP levels remain high as long as the inflammation or tissue damage persists and then decrease rapidly. The half life time of CRP is 19 hours under all conditions, which shows the synthesis rate alone is responsible for the actual serum concentration. [18]

4. Serial CRP determinations are of high sensitivity in diagnosis of neonatal sepsis

CRP passes the placenta only in very low quantities, therefore, any elevation in the neonate always represents endogenous synthesis. [19] De novo hepatic synthesis starts very rapidly after a single stimulus with serum concentrations rising above 5 mg/l by about 6 hours and peaking around 48 hours. [20]

In diagnosis of early onset sepsis previous studies reported on widely differing sensitivities and specificities of CRP ranging from 29% to 100% and from 6% to 100%, respectively. [11,

21, 22] These extreme variations are a result of different reference-values, test methodologies, patient characteristics and inclusion criteria, number of samples taken, and sampling time. Furthermore, definitions of sepsis widely differ between studies making serious comparisons hardly possible.

The sensitivity of CRP is known to be the lowest during the early stages of infection. [23-25] For a single CRP determination at the time of first sepsis evaluation the sensitivity and specificity range from 22% to 69% and from 90% to 96%, respectively. [23, 24, 26-29] Similar results were reported for cord blood CRP. Even with low cut-off values being used [1 to 5 mg/l) sensitivities and specificities ranged from 22 to 74% and from 78 to 97%, respectively. [30-33] Thus, a single normal value at the initial sepsis work-up is not sufficient to rule out an infection [11].

On the other hand a raised CRP is not necessarily diagnostic for sepsis, as elevations may as well occur due to the physiologic rise after birth or non infection associated conditions (see below). Therefore, concerns were raised about the reliability of CRP during the early stage of the disease being neither able to diagnose nor to rule out an infection with certainty. [23]

Benitz et al. [23] found that the sensitivity in the diagnosis of culture proven early onset sepsis increased from 35% at the initial sepsis work-up to 79% and 89% when CRP determination was performed on the two following days. In a large series of 689 neonates (187 with sepsis) Pourcyrous et al. [24] reported a higher sensitivity for CRP levels determined at least 12 hours after the initial evaluation compared to the first value (54% vs. 74%). In general the sensitivity substantially increases with serial determinations 24 to 48 hours after the onset of symptoms, and several studies reported on sensitivities and specificities ranging from 78% to 98% and from 81% to 97%, respectively. [11, 21, 23-27, 34]

Some authors have suggested that serial determinations may be useful for identification of infants who do not have a bacterial infection as well: Two consecutive CRP values <10 mg/l carry a 99% negative predictive value in accurately identifying infants not infected. [6, 21, 23, 35-37] At 48 h after onset of symptoms with at least two normal CRP values and negative blood cultures infection can be ruled out and antibiotics can be stopped. [38]

Similarly, serial CRP measurements can be helpful in monitoring the response to treatment in infected neonates, to determine the duration of antibiotic therapy, and to recognize possible complications. [21, 25, 39] In a cohort of 60 neonates with early onset sepsis Ehl et al. [40] demonstrated that after initiation of a successful antibiotic therapy CRP values further increased, peaking and consecutively decreasing after 16 hours. A CRP level that returned again to the normal range may indicate that the duration of antibiotic treatment has been sufficient allowing discontinuation of antibiotics. [35]

5. CRP values can be elevated in non-infectious conditions

In adults, elevated CRP concentration was described in a large variety of disorders apart from bacterial, viral, and fungal infections including burns, surgery, rheumatic disorders, malignancies, and vasculitis. [20]

In neonates, non infection associated elevation of CRP was described in conditions of maternal and perinatal distress, neonatal hypoxia, and tissue damage. Several authors have described links of CRP to maternal fever, stressful delivery, prolonged rupture of membranes and/or prolonged labor, asphyxia, meconium aspiration syndrome, intraventricular hemorrhage, pneumothorax, and tissue injury. [19, 24, 34, 41-49] (see table 1)

-Perinatal asphyxia/ shock [34, 41, 43, 45] -Maternal fever during labor [41, 42] -Prolonged rupture of membranes [41-45] -Stressful delivery or fetal distress [19, 41, 43] -Prolonged labor [42, 44, 46] -Clinically silent meconium aspiration[42] -Surfactant application [48, 64] -Intra-ventricular hemorrhage[34, 43] -Pneumo-thorax.[34] -Tissue injury[24]

Table 1. Non-infectious conditions associated with increased CRP values during the first days of life.

However, the issue on non-infectious CRP elevations in the neonate is not undisputed. Different studies gave to some extent inconsistent results and conditions that some authors described being associated with CRP elevation were not found in other analyses. The earliest descriptions on non infectious conditions influencing CRP derive from simple observations that elevated values in not infected infants might be connected to coincidental non-infectious conditions, though no statistical confirmation is given.

Few investigations were performed on the association of CRP with non infectious conditions in healthy neonates. Chiesa et al. evaluated conditions influencing what constitutes normal CRP values in healthy neonates. In their analysis on 148 healthy term or near term neonates they identified low 5-minute Apgar score and premature rupture of membranes being significantly associated with CRP response at birth and pregnancy induced hypertension with CRP response at 24 hours of life. [45] In a similarly selected cohort of 421 healthy neonates including 200 premature infants they confirmed an association with the time of ruptured membranes and added duration of active labor, prenatal steroids, and intrapartum antimicrobial prophylaxis as variables that had a significant effect on CRP concentrations when adjusted for gestational age, gender, and sampling time. [44]

The current literature suggests that CRP may be elevated in some non-infectious conditions, of which some may per se clinically mimic a bacterial infection as well. Thus, the up to date available information lacks in robust evidence to support a claim that withholding antibiotics may be justified in infants with raised CRP in the above mentioned conditions.

6. CRP performance in diagnosis of neonatal sepsis and baseline CRP concentrations differ between term and preterm neonates

Even though advances in neonatal intensive care have led to increasing preterm birth rates and survival rates, the influences of prematurity on laboratory test results are poorly understood and have not been assessed systematically. This is also true for CRP, which is one of the most extensively studied infection markers in the neonatal period. Reports on the influence of gestational age on kinetics of CRP in infected and uninfected infants are limited:

Turner et al. [50] demonstrated an association of gestational age with the magnitude of clinically relevant CRP responses during the first seven days after birth. In case of a clinically relevant CRP rise >10 mg/l the proportion of a pronounced response >60 mg/l increased with gestational age from 8% in newborns from 24 to 27 weeks to 25% in newborns from 40 to 41 weeks.

Several other authors have contributed to the growing body of evidence further supporting the difference in CRP response to infection between term and preterm infants. In a cohort of 348 infants Kawamura et al. [25] reported a lower sensitivity of CRP in the diagnosis of neonatal sepsis in preterm compared to term newborns (61.5% vs. 75%).

Doellner et al. [51] described a significantly lower CRP increase induced by infection in preterm compared to term infants. In their cohort of 42 newborns with either culture proven or probable sepsis infants with a gestational age less than 35 weeks had lower CRP values and lower CRP peak values compared to infants with a gestational age greater than 35 weeks (CRP values 0 vs 18 mg/l, CRP peak values 15 vs 52 mg/l).

We have recently reported on a lower CRP response to infection in preterm compared to term newborns with a lower sensitivity (53% vs. 86%), lower median values (9 vs. 18.5 mg/l), and a lower area under the receiver operating characteristics curve (0.799 vs. 0.890). [48]

What might explain the observed differences of CRP values between term and preterm newborns? One fact might be the differences in pre- and postnatal care regarding more frequent prophylactic antibiotic treatment in preterm infants and their mothers during birth. Timing of blood sampling might be another critical point being possibly earlier in preterm newborns. CRP is thought to play an important role in innate immunity, as an early defence system against infections. As far as the endogenous immune response depends on gestational age CRP responses might be lower due to a less mature immunological system of the preterm newborn.

Table 2 gives an overview on current literature on the association of CRP kinetics with gestational age and/or birth weight.

For neonates, assessment of laboratory tests occurs within a complex context of prenatal growth and neonatal development. [52] Though the current literature reveals some minor disagreement on the effect of gestational age on CRP there is a body of growing evidence suggesting that the so far reported characteristics of CRP may not be as suitable for the use in preterm as in term newborns. Their baseline CRP values may be lower and their response to infection less distinct. Prematurity of the organ systems and maturational changes in the immune system might result in a more distinct CRP response to delivery in uninfected newborns and to bacterial invasion in infected newborns. The few studies so far addressing this issue suggest that the diagnostic accuracy of CRP in preterm infants may benefit from a re-evaluation of the reference intervals in this age group. [25, 44, 48, 51]

Author	Cohort			
Diagnostic accuracy		Sensitivity (%)		
Kawamura et al. [25]	348 neonates with suspicion of infection	61.5 vs. 75		(preterm vs. term neonates)
Hofer et al. [48]	532 uninfected and infected neonates	53 vs. 86		(preterm vs. term neonates at 8 mg/l cut-off value)
		Highest sensitivity in preterm infants at the cut-off 5.5 mg/l (74%) and at 10.5 mg/l in term infants (86%)		
CRP concentration		median (mg/l)	peak (mg/l)	
Doellner et al. [51]	42 neonates with probable or proven sepsis	0 vs. 18	15 vs. 52	(<35 weeks vs. ≥35 weeks)
Hofer et al. [48]	499 uninfected neonates	0.2 vs. 2.0	9.0 vs. 26.2	(preterm vs. term neonates)
	33 neonates with proven sepsis	9.0 vs. 18.5	40.4 vs. 98.6	(preterm vs. term neonates)
Ishibashi et al. [46]	110 uninfected symptomatic neonates	Gestational age and birth weight significantly influence hsCRP concentration within 48 hours after birth. Infants with low gestational age and low birth weight had lower hsCRP concentration (p=.013 and .024, respectively).		
Chiesa et al. [44]	421 healthy neonates	By regression analysis mean CRP increased by 6% per week gestational age at delivery (p<.01) and per 2.4% per 100 g increase in birth weight (p<.01)		
Turner et al. [50]	3574 neonates	In case of a clinically relevant CRP rise >10 mg/l, the proportion of a pronounced response >60 mg/l increased with gestational age from 8% in newborns from 24 to 27 weeks to 25% in newborns from 40 to 41 weeks.		

Table 2. Overview on current literature on the difference in CRP kinetics between term and preterm neonates.

7. Performance of CRP in diagnosis of neonatal sepsis can further be enhanced by combining it with early sensitive markers

An important limitation of CRP is the low sensitivity during the early phases of sepsis. By then values are often still normal, though the consequences of the bacterial invasion are already apparent and a delay of the initiation of antibiotic therapy may be associated with an adverse outcome. CRP takes ten to twelve hours to significantly change after the onset of infection. [6] Earlier in the inflammatory cascade activated macrophages release pro-inflammatory cytokines (IL-1, IL-6, TNF-α) and growth factors (IL-3, CSFs) inducing the hepatic synthesis of acute-phase-reactants and the activation of neutrophils. The increase of cytokines therefore precedes the changes of CRP. Of the many mediators studied, much attention has been focused on IL6, IL8, and TNF-α.

IL-6 increases rapidly after the bacterial invasion and was demonstrated to have a high sensitivity during the early stages of sepsis (80%-100%) even when determined from umbilical cord blood (87%-100%). [29, 53) However, a short half life caused by plasma protein binding, hepatic clearance, and inactivation results in a rapid normalization of serum levels and a decrease of sensitivity during the later course of the disease, even though the infection persists. IL-8 and TNF-α have very similar characteristics and kinetic properties to IL-6. Both are pro-inflammatory cytokines predominantly produced by activated phagocytes in response to systemic infection and inflammation. [53] While studies report on a reliable diagnostic accuracy of IL-8 with a sensitivity of 69%-100%, the usefulness of TNF-α as a diagnostic marker has not been found to be as good as either IL-6 or IL-8. [53, 54]

Similar to CRP procalcitonin is another important acute-phase reactant produced by monocytes and hepatocytes. It has the advantage of increasing more rapidly after contact to bacterial endotoxin with levels rising after four hours and peaking at six to eight hours [55] In a recent meta-analysis the sensitivity and specificity in the diagnosis of early onset sepsis were 76% (range 68–82%) and 76% (60–87%). [56] Though the sensitivity during the early stages of sepsis may be superior to CRP, the significant rapid variations of basal levels after birth, the increase after non-infectious conditions such as asphyxia, maternal pre-eclampsia, and intracranial hemorrhage,[57] and the need for several different cut-off values with changing neonatal age, have limited its diffusion as an early marker in comparison to CRP.

Specific leukocyte cell surface antigens are known to be expressed in substantial quantities after inflammatory cells are activated by bacteria or their cellular products. [62] From the amount of surface markers studied neutrophil CD11b and CD64 appear most promising for diagnosis of neonatal sepsis. CD11b expression increases considerably within a few minutes after the inflammatory cells come into contact with bacteria and endotoxins. [58, 59] The sensitivity and specificity of CD11b for diagnosing early onset neonatal sepsis are 86–100% and 100% respectively. [7, 53] CD64 has a sensitivity ranging between 81% and 96% and a NPV between 89% and 97%. [60] Though promising, estimation of cell surface markers is limited by the need for sophisticated equipment and the need to process blood samples rapidly before neutrophils die from apoptosis or the surface antigens are down regulated. [61]

Despite the favorable claims by many studies, many of these diagnostic markers fail to meet the stringent demands required for clinical practice. High costs, limited availability of specimens at the appropriate time, and complexity of the assay methods all limit the clinical applicability. More importantly, the relatively small sample size in most studies, the lack of clear reference values for many diagnostic markers still prohibit the use of most of these parameters in clinical practice.

Sensitivity is low during the early phase of infection. The performance of serial determinations 24 to 48 hours after the onset of symptoms is recommended, as it clearly improves diagnostic accuracy.
CRP is particularly useful for ruling out an infection and for monitoring the response to treatment and guiding the duration of the antibiotic therapy. Two consecutive values <10 mg/l determined more than 24 hours apart identify infants unlikely to be infected or in whom infection has resolved.
CRP values undergo a physiological 3-day-rise after birth and non-infectious confounders such as meconium aspiration syndrome and perinatal maternal risk conditions may elevate CRP values in otherwise healthy newborns.
Preterm neonates have lower baseline CRP values and a lower CRP response to infection in compared to term newborns.
Data on non infectious CRP elevations in otherwise healthy newborns are inconsistent and does currently not allow drawing recommendations on the continuation or withdrawal of antibiotics in these infants.
Up to date the most used cut-off value is 10 mg/l irrespective of the gestational and postnatal age of the neonate. Cut-off values adapted to the gestational and postnatal age may better reflect neonatal physiology.
In order to compensate for the diagnostic weakness during the early phases of infection initial CRP determination should be combined with determination of early and sensitive markers. Suitable markers include but are not limited to PCT, IL6, and IL8. Many further parameters may provide similar good results but are not yet sufficiently examined to be applied to clinical practice.

Table 3. CRP facts.

At the moment none of the described current diagnostic markers are sensitive and specific enough to influence the judgment to withhold antimicrobial treatment independent of the clinical findings. Efforts were done to improve diagnostic accuracy by combining multiple markers in order to further enhance the diagnostic accuracy of these mediators in identifying infected cases.

CRP has been investigated in combination with a variety of "new" infection markers including cytokines, surface markers, and other acute-phase-reactants with promising results. Especially the combination with an early sensitive marker such as PCT, IL6, IL8, CD11b, and CD64 increases the sensitivity to values between 90% and 100% in most studies.

8. Do special subpopulations need special CRP reference values?

Especially in the early neonatal period, many physiological and metabolic processes are in change and differ from every later moment in life. These changes affect several laboratory parameters as well and many reference values and serum kinetics substantially differ to later periods. [62]

Reliable reference values are crucial for obtaining an adequate diagnostic accuracy. Upper limits for CRP during the first days of life have mainly been established from uninfected but symptomatic neonates. The cut-off values reported in the literature range from 1,5mg/l to 20 mg/l with thus wide ranging sensitivities and specificities. [11, 63] The up to date most used upper limit for CRP during the first days of life of 10 mg/l has been established in 1987 by Mathers and Pohlandt. [28] One decade later, Benitz et al. evaluated CRP levels in 1002 episodes of suspected early onset sepsis and confirmed the value being an appropriate threshold level. [23]

Use of CRP in the first few days after birth is complicated by a nonspecific rise primarily related to the stress of delivery. [11, 45] This rise of CRP starts shortly after birth and peaks with 13 mg/l in term and 11 mg/l in preterm newborns during the second and third day of life, respectively. [44] These observations raise concern about the static cut-off value not reflecting the physiologic kinetics of CRP after birth. In view of the physiologic dynamics of CRP during the first days after birth and the influence of gestational age on its response to infection, it appears reasonable to reconsider this static cut-off value and evaluate the possible advantages of the introduction of dynamic reference values. However, the current literature lacks sufficient evidence to make recommendations for the use in clinical practice.

9. Conclusion

CRP is one of the most widely available, most studied, and most used laboratory tests for neonatal bacterial infection and despite the continuing emergence of new infection markers it still plays a central role in the diagnosis of early onset sepsis of the neonate. CRP has the advantage of being well characterized in numerous studies and the extensive knowledge on its properties and limitations makes it safer compared to other, newer markers. Still, further research is needed on the topics of the influence of gestational age on CRP kinetics in infection, non-infectious confounders, and the evaluation of dynamic and gestational age dependent reference values.

Author details

Nora Hofer

Research Unit for Neonatal Infectious Diseases and Epidemiology, Medical University of Graz, Austria

Wilhelm Müller

Division of Neonatology, Department of Pediatrics and Adolescent Medicine, Medical University of Graz, Austria

Bernhard Resch

Research Unit for Neonatal Infectious Diseases and Epidemiology, Medical University of Graz, Austria

Division of Neonatology, Department of Pediatrics and Adolescent Medicine, Medical University of Graz, Austria

10. References

[1] Fanaroff AA, Stoll BJ, Wright LL, Carlo WA, Ehrenkranz RA, Stark AR, et al. Trends in neonatal morbidity and mortality for very low birthweight infants. American Journal of Obstetrics and Gynecology. 2007;196(2):147.e1-8-.e1-8.

[2] Remington JS, Klein JO. Developmental immunology and role of host defenses in neonatal susceptibility. In: Remington JS, Klein, editors. Infectious Diseases of the Fetus and Newborn Infant. Philadelphia: Saunders; 1990. p. 17-67.

[3] Murray BE. Can antibiotic resistance be controlled? The New England Journal of Medicine. 1994;330(17):1229-30.

[4] Hotchkiss RS, Karl IE. The pathophysiology and treatment of sepsis. The New England Journal of Medicine. 2003;348(2):138-50.

[5] Russell JA. Management of sepsis. The New England Journal of Medicine. 2006;355(16):1699-713.

[6] Chirico G, Loda C. Laboratory aid to the diagnosis and therapy of infection in the neonate. Pediatric Reports. 2011;3(1):e1-e.

[7] Mishra UK, Jacobs SE, Doyle LW, Garland SM. Newer approaches to the diagnosis of early onset neonatal sepsis. Archives of Disease in Childhood Fetal and Neonatal Edition. 2006;91(3):F208-12-F-12.

[8] Ng PC, Li K, Leung TF, Wong RPO, Li G, Chui KM, et al. Early prediction of sepsis-induced disseminated intravascular coagulation with interleukin-10, interleukin-6, and RANTES in preterm infants. Clinical Chemistry. 2006;52(6):1181-9.

[9] Tillett WS, Francis T. Serological Reactions in Pneumonia with a Non-Protein Somatic Fraction of Pneumococcus. The Journal of Experimental Medicine. 1930;52(4):561-71.

[10] Pepys MB. C-reactive protein fifty years on. Lancet. 1981;1(8221):653-7.

[11] Jaye DL, Waites KB. Clinical applications of C-reactive protein in pediatrics. The Pediatric Infectious Disease Journal. 1997;16(8):735-46.

[12] Volanakis JE. Human C-reactive protein: expression, structure, and function. Molecular Immunology. 2001;38(2-3):189-97.

[13] Du Clos TW. Function of C-reactive protein. Annals of Medicine. 2000;32(4):274-8.

[14] Weinhold B, Rüther U. Interleukin-6-dependent and -independent regulation of the human C-reactive protein gene. The Biochemical Journal. 1997;327 (Pt 2):425-9.

[15] Shine B, de Beer FC, Pepys MB. Solid phase radioimmunoassays for human C-reactive protein. Clinica Chimica Acta; International Journal of Clinical Chemistry. 1981;117(1):13-23.

[16] Rifai N, Ridker PM. Population distributions of C-reactive protein in apparently healthy men and women in the United States: implication for clinical interpretation. Clinical Chemistry. 2003;49(4):666-9.

[17] Imhof A, Fröhlich M, Loewel H, Helbecque N, Woodward M, Amouyel P, et al. Distributions of C-reactive protein measured by high-sensitivity assays in apparently healthy men and women from different populations in Europe. Clinical Chemistry. 2003;49(4):669-72.

[18] Vigushin DM, Pepys MB, Hawkins PN. Metabolic and scintigraphic studies of radioiodinated human C-reactive protein in health and disease. The Journal of Clinical Investigation. 1993;91(4):1351-7.

[19] Kääpä P, Koistinen E. Maternal and neonatal C-reactive protein after interventions during delivery. Acta Obstetricia Et Gynecologica Scandinavica. 1993;72(7):543-6.

[20] Pepys MB, Hirschfield GM. C-reactive protein: a critical update. The Journal of Clinical Investigation. 2003;111(12):1805-12.

[21] Hengst JM. The role of C-reactive protein in the evaluation and management of infants with suspected sepsis. Advances in Neonatal Care: Official Journal of the National Association of Neonatal Nurses. 2003;3(1):3-13.

[22] Fowlie PW, Schmidt B. Diagnostic tests for bacterial infection from birth to 90 days--a systematic review. Archives of Disease in Childhood Fetal and Neonatal Edition. 1998;78(2):F92-8-F-8.

[23] Benitz WE, Han MY, Madan A, Ramachandra P. Serial serum C-reactive protein levels in the diagnosis of neonatal infection. Pediatrics. 1998;102(4):E41-E.

[24] Pourcyrous M, Bada HS, Korones SB, Baselski V, Wong SP. Significance of serial C-reactive protein responses in neonatal infection and other disorders. Pediatrics. 1993;92(3):431-5.

[25] Kawamura M, Nishida H. The usefulness of serial C-reactive protein measurement in managing neonatal infection. Acta Paediatrica (Oslo, Norway: 1992). 1995;84(1):10-3.

[26] Laborada G, Rego M, Jain A, Guliano M, Stavola J, Ballabh P, et al. Diagnostic value of cytokines and C-reactive protein in the first 24 hours of neonatal sepsis. American Journal of Perinatology. 2003;20(8):491-501.

[27] Wagle S, Grauaug A, Kohan R, Evans SF. C-reactive protein as a diagnostic tool of sepsis in very immature babies. Journal of Paediatrics and Child Health. 1994;30(1):40-4.

[28] Mathers NJ, Pohlandt F. Diagnostic audit of C-reactive protein in neonatal infection. European Journal of Pediatrics. 1987;146(2):147-51.

[29] Resch B, Gusenleitner W, Müller WD. Procalcitonin and interleukin-6 in the diagnosis of early-onset sepsis of the neonate. Acta Paediatrica (Oslo, Norway: 1992). 2003;92(2):243-5.

[30] Joram N, Boscher C, Denizot S, Loubersac V, Winer N, Roze JC, et al. Umbilical cord blood procalcitonin and C reactive protein concentrations as markers for early diagnosis of very early onset neonatal infection. Archives of Disease in Childhood Fetal and Neonatal Edition. 2006;91(1):F65-6-F-6.

[31] Kordek A, Giedrys-Kalemba S, Pawlus B, Podraza W, Czajka R. Umbilical cord blood serum procalcitonin concentration in the diagnosis of early neonatal infection. Journal of Perinatology: Official Journal of the California Perinatal Association. 2003;23(2):148-53.

[32] Kordek A, Hałasa M, Podraza W. Early detection of an early onset infection in the neonate based on measurements of procalcitonin and C-reactive protein concentrations in cord blood. Clinical Chemistry and Laboratory Medicine: CCLM / FESCC. 2008;46(8):1143-8.

[33] Chiesa C, Pellegrini G, Panero A, Osborn JF, Signore F, Assumma M, et al. C-reactive protein, interleukin-6, and procalcitonin in the immediate postnatal period: influence of illness severity, risk status, antenatal and perinatal complications, and infection. Clinical Chemistry. 2003;49(1):60-8.

[34] Berger C, Uehlinger J, Ghelfi D, Blau N, Fanconi S. Comparison of C-reactive protein and white blood cell count with differential in neonates at risk for septicaemia. European Journal of Pediatrics. 1995;154(2):138-44.
[35] Ehl S, Gering B, Bartmann P, Högel J, Pohlandt F. C-reactive protein is a useful marker for guiding duration of antibiotic therapy in suspected neonatal bacterial infection. Pediatrics. 1997;99(2):216-21.
[36] Bomela HN, Ballot DE, Cory BJ, Cooper PA. Use of C-reactive protein to guide duration of empiric antibiotic therapy in suspected early neonatal sepsis. The Pediatric Infectious Disease Journal. 2000;19(6):531-5.
[37] Philip AG, Mills PC. Use of C-reactive protein in minimizing antibiotic exposure: experience with infants initially admitted to a well-baby nursery. Pediatrics. 2000;106(1):E4-E.
[38] McWilliam S, Riordan A. How to use: C-reactive protein. Archives of Disease in Childhood Education and Practice Edition. 2010;95(2):55-8.
[39] Franz AR, Steinbach G, Kron M, Pohlandt F. Reduction of unnecessary antibiotic therapy in newborn infants using interleukin-8 and C-reactive protein as markers of bacterial infections. Pediatrics. 1999;104(3 Pt 1):447-53.
[40] Ehl S, Gehring B, Pohlandt F. A detailed analysis of changes in serum C-reactive protein levels in neonates treated for bacterial infection. European Journal of Pediatrics. 1999;158(3):238-42.
[41] Ainbender E, Cabatu EE, Guzman DM, Sweet AY. Serum C-reactive protein and problems of newborn infants. The Journal of Pediatrics. 1982;101(3):438-40.
[42] Mathai E, Christopher U, Mathai M, Jana AK, Rose D, Bergstrom S. Is C-reactive protein level useful in differentiating infected from uninfected neonates among those at risk of infection? Indian Pediatrics. 2004;41(9):895-900.
[43] Forest JC, Larivière F, Dolcé P, Masson M, Nadeau L. C-reactive protein as biochemical indicator of bacterial infection in neonates. Clinical Biochemistry. 1986;19(3):192-4.
[44] Chiesa C, Natale F, Pascone R, Osborn JF, Pacifico L, Bonci E, et al. C reactive protein and procalcitonin: reference intervals for preterm and term newborns during the early neonatal period. Clinica Chimica Acta; International Journal of Clinical Chemistry. 2011;412(11-12):1053-9.
[45] Chiesa C, Signore F, Assumma M, Buffone E, Tramontozzi P, Osborn JF, et al. Serial measurements of C-reactive protein and interleukin-6 in the immediate postnatal period: reference intervals and analysis of maternal and perinatal confounders. Clinical Chemistry. 2001;47(6):1016-22.
[46] Ishibashi M, Takemura Y, Ishida H, Watanabe K, Kawai T. C-reactive protein kinetics in newborns: application of a high-sensitivity analytic method in its determination. Clinical Chemistry. 2002;48(7):1103-6.
[47] Dyck RF, Bingham W, Tan L, Rogers SL. Serum levels of C-reactive protein in neonatal respiratory distress syndrome. Clinical Pediatrics. 1984;23(7):381-3.
[48] Hofer N, Müller W, Resch B. Non-infectious conditions and gestational age influence C-reactive protein values in newborns during the first 3 days of life. Clinical Chemistry and Laboratory Medicine: CCLM / FESCC. 2011;49(2):297-302.

[49] Pourcyrous M, Bada HS, Korones SB, Barrett FF, Jennings W, Lockey T. Acute phase reactants in neonatal bacterial infection. Journal of Perinatology: Official Journal of the California Perinatal Association. 1991;11(4):319-25.

[50] Turner MA, Power S, Emmerson AJB. Gestational age and the C reactive protein response. Archives of Disease in Childhood Fetal and Neonatal Edition. 2004;89(3):F272-3-F-3.

[51] Doellner H, Arntzen KJ, Haereid PE, Aag S, Austgulen R. Interleukin-6 concentrations in neonates evaluated for sepsis. The Journal of Pediatrics. 1998;132(2):295-9.

[52] Chiesa C, Osborn JF, Pacifico L, Natale F, De Curtis M. Gestational- and age-specific CRP reference intervals in the newborn. Clinica Chimica Acta; International Journal of Clinical Chemistry. 2011;412(19-20):1889-90.

[53] Ng PC. Diagnostic markers of infection in neonates. Archives of Disease in Childhood Fetal and Neonatal Edition. 2004;89(3):F229-35-F-35.

[54] Malik A, Hui CPS, Pennie RA, Kirpalani H. Beyond the complete blood cell count and C-reactive protein: a systematic review of modern diagnostic tests for neonatal sepsis. Archives of Pediatrics & Adolescent Medicine. 2003;157(6):511-6.

[55] Dandona P, Nix D, Wilson MF, Aljada A, Love J, Assicot M, et al. Procalcitonin increase after endotoxin injection in normal subjects. The Journal of Clinical Endocrinology and Metabolism. 1994;79(6):1605-8.

[56] Vouloumanou EK, Plessa E, Karageorgopoulos DE, Mantadakis E, Falagas ME. Serum procalcitonin as a diagnostic marker for neonatal sepsis: a systematic review and meta-analysis. Intensive Care Medicine. 2011;37(5):747-62.

[57] Lam HS, Ng PC. Biochemical markers of neonatal sepsis. Pathology. 2008;40(2):141-8.

[58] Simms HH, D'Amico R. Lipopolysaccharide induces intracytoplasmic migration of the polymorphonuclear leukocyte CD11b/CD18 receptor. Shock (Augusta, Ga). 1995;3(3):196-203.

[59] Lehr HA, Krombach F, Münzing S, Bodlaj R, Glaubitt SI, Seiffge D, et al. In vitro effects of oxidized low density lipoprotein on CD11b/CD18 and L-selectin presentation on neutrophils and monocytes with relevance for the in vivo situation. The American Journal of Pathology. 1995;146(1):218-27.

[60] Ng PC, Li G, Chui KM, Chu WCW, Li K, Wong RPO, et al. Neutrophil CD64 is a sensitive diagnostic marker for early-onset neonatal infection. Pediatric Research. 2004;56(5):796-803.

[61] Haque KN. Neonatal Sepsis in the Very Low Birth Weight Preterm Infants: Part 2: Review of Definition, Diagnosis and Management. Journal of Medical Sciences. 2010;1(3):11-7.

[62] Van Lente F, Pippenger CE. The pediatric acute care laboratory. Pediatric Clinics of North America. 1987;34(1):231-46.

[63] Chiesa C, Panero A, Osborn JF, Simonetti AF, Pacifico L. Diagnosis of neonatal sepsis: a clinical and laboratory challenge. Clinical Chemistry. 2004;50(2):279-87.

[64] Kukkonen AK, Virtanen M, Järvenpää AL, Pokela ML, Ikonen S, Fellman V. Randomized trial comparing natural and synthetic surfactant: increased infection rate after natural surfactant? Acta Paediatrica (Oslo, Norway: 1992). 2000;89(5):556-61.

Chapter 5

The Role of Immature Granulocyte Count and Immature Myeloid Information in the Diagnosis of Neonatal Sepsis

Christina Cimenti, Wolfgang Erwa, Wilhelm Müller and Bernhard Resch

Additional information is available at the end of the chapter

http://dx.doi.org/10.5772/54531

1. Introduction

Although diagnostic and therapeutic approaches to neonatal sepsis considerably progressed over the last decades, distinguishing infected from non-infected patients still remains a major challenge, especially in the early phase of disease when symptoms are often subtle and unspecific. Development and application of potent antibiotic medication and the advances in neonatal care could improve treatment but incidence of neonatal sepsis is still high. Compared to an incidence rate ranging from 1.5 to 3.5 per 1000 for neonatal early onset sepsis (EOS) and up to 6 per 1000 live births for late onset sepsis (LOS) in developed countries, the reported incidence of neonatal sepsis varies from 7.1 to 38 per 1000 live births in Asia and from 6.5 to 23 per 1000 live births in Africa (Vergnano et al., 2005). The physiologic immature state of the immune system and reduced levels of preformed maternal antibodies in preterm infants together with organ immaturity and a lower expression of major histocompatibility complex (MHC) class II antigens on monocytes contribute to a disturbed equilibrium of pro- and anti-inflammatory factors resulting in a reduced immune defence making the preterm infant more susceptible for sepsis and its short and long term complications (Azizia et al., 2012; Stoll et al., 2004). Prospective data collection of 16 participating centers of the National Institute of Child Health and Human Development Neonatal Research Network revealed a declining incidence of blood culture proven EOS from 19.3 per 1000 in 1991-93 to 15.4 per 1000 live births in 1998-2000 among very low birth weight (VLBW) infants, whereas the incidence of late-onset septicemia was 22% and remained essentially unchanged over the observed period of time. However, the potentially life threatening character of EOS is reflected by high mortality rates reaching between 1.6% in nonblack term infants and 37% in preterm infants with VLBW (Fanaroff et al., 2007; Weston et al., 2011). Infants in this study without EOS showed a significantly reduced mortality risk of 13%.

Considering these data it is comprehensible that many neonatologists hazard the consequences of possibly unnecessary exposure to antimicrobial agents in neonates suspected for sepsis with unspecific symptoms and uncertain infectious state to avoid fatal outcome caused by a delay in treatment. The above-mentioned declined incidence of EOS was mainly caused by a change in the pathogen distribution showing a decline in group B streptococcus (GBS) sepsis but an increase in Escherichia coli sepsis with a rate of 85% of ampicillin resistance (Fanaroff et al., 2007). As the use of broad-spectrum antimicrobial agents like the combination of ampicillin and an aminoglycoside is considered as the optimal treatment of infants with suspected EOS (Polin, 2012), the progressively increasing burden of antimicrobial resistance would actually require a more targeted drug therapy in the future to confine human and economic costs. The often unspecific early symptoms and the potential rapid deterioration necessitate early identification of patients at risk. This should help to avoid a delay in treatment and could prevent further complications. On the other hand, overtreatment of newborn infants with maternal risk factors and uncertain infectious status suspected for sepsis could also be reduced helping to avoid prescription of unnecessary prophylactic broad-spectrum antibiotic medication, to restrain the development of antimicrobial resistance, exposing the patients to possible severe adverse effects and help to increase cost effectiveness.

1.1. Diagnostic approaches to neonatal sepsis

Despite a myriad number of scientific studies evaluating the performance of laboratory markers, risk scores, and clinical features in neonatal sepsis, the search for a perfect diagnostic test with high accuracy and reliability still seems to be a quest for the holy grail (Briggs et al., 2000). Still, no single laboratory parameter and none of the newly created clinical risk scores are generally accepted to define the diagnosis of sepsis in its early course with 100% accuracy and confidence (Fowlie & Schmidt, 1998; Rodwell et al., 1988). A systematic review of the literature of 194 studies reporting on different diagnostic tests to predict the presence or absence of bacterial infection in infants up to 90 days of age generally described a poor methodological quality (Fowlie & Schmidt, 1998). Even in rigorous studies the accuracy of the tests showed enormous variation and the diagnostic value was considered as limited in this population (Fowlie & Schmidt, 1998). Although blood culture is considered as the gold standard to confirm the diagnosis of sepsis, this method has its limitations in a neonatal - especially in a preterm – population (Chiesa et al., 2004; Fowlie & Schmidt, 1998). In a study to determine the minimum required blood volume to detect bacteremia Schelonka found that a 0.5 mL blood sample –as commonly obtained in neonatal intensive care units (NICU) - is insufficient to obtain sensitive results when the colony count is less than 4/mL. This is of special interest as it has been shown that low-level bacteremia is common in infants less than two months of age accounting up to 68% (Kellogg et al., 1997; Schelonka et al., 1996). Furthermore false negative results can be obtained due to the presence of antimicrobial agents in the blood because of an early onset of treatment based on empirically decision making representing a regular practice in clinical routine (Fowlie & Schmidt, 1998). Because blood culture bottles require sufficient incubation time, results are delayed and can normally be expected within three days, whereas in infants up to an age of 72 hours blood cultures require a longer incubation time. In a retrospective observational study comprising more than 2900 neonates the median time to positivity of blood cultures was significantly shorter in Gram negative (11.2 hours; 8.5-15.7) compared to Gram positive organisms (23.6 hours; 15.3-4.6). These findings could have important clinical implications to optimize antimicrobial therapy. The authors suggest targeting only for Gram positive germs when the blood culture is still negative after 48 hours and to cease treatment in well-being infants without clinical and laboratory signs of infection after 72 hours when blood culture remains sterile (Guerti et al., 2011).

Generally, blood culture-proven EOS has been described as quite uncommon in a large multicenter investigation of neonates with VLBW occurring in only 1.9%. Whereas almost 50% of the study population was characterized for sepsis because of clinical signs, in 98% blood culture reports revealed negative results, but antibiotic treatment was continued fearing false negative results possibly due to maternal antibiotic medication (Stoll et al., 1996). A high rate of failed detection of bacterial growth in blood cultures of VLBW neonates between 27% and 92% could possibly be explained by a transient or intermittent bacteremia as sepsis is known to be a dynamic process (Haque, 2010). Beyond that, interpreting results when organisms are of low or questionable virulence as pathogen or possible contamination- frequently occurring during blood collection (Pourcyrous et al., 1993)- is often difficult.

1.1.1. The White blood cell count (WBC) as primary diagnostic tool in neonatal sepsis

Although several studies have shown a poor predictive value performing a single WBC as a screening method in asymptomatic neonates with infectious risk factors or later on culture proven sepsis (Ottolini et al., 2003; Rozycki et al., 1987), the assessment of a complete blood cell count (CBC) is usually performed as a routine method to evaluate newborns at risk. The recent introduction of several new parameters to the routine CBC with white blood differential performed by automated hematology analyzer have enabled quantification of cells which were previously solely classified as abnormal flags (Briggs et al., 2003). This refers mainly to the compartment of immature neutrophil granulocytes (IG) which have been detected in various conditions including later stage of pregnancy, steroid therapy, cancer, trauma, or myeloproliferative diseases (Briggs, 2009). They have been considered as helpful early indicators of infectious conditions (Buttarello & Plebani, 2008; Rodwell et al., 1988) and have a long clinical tradition in the diagnosis of bacterial sepsis in neonates (Akenzua et al., 1974).

A commonly used index to comprise the fraction of IG in the clinical practice is the IT (immature-to-total-neutrophil)-ratio which is defined as the proportion of the number of immature cells including blasts, band cells, myelocytes, and metamyelocytes to the number of mature neutrophil cells. It is a manual count usually determined by a peripheral blood smear. Already more than three decades ago elevation of IT-ratio was considered to be a useful aid in the diagnosis of neonatal bacterial sepsis. The authors suggested that the higher the degree of elevated IT-ratio was, the higher was the risk of bone marrow depletion and death from sepsis (Christensen et al., 1981).

In a retrospective multicenter cohort analysis including 166092 neonates with suspected EOS admitted to 293 NICUs in the United States low WBC counts, low absolute neutrophil counts, and high IT-ratios were associated with increasing odds of infection. Elevated IT-ratios of >0.2, >0.25, and >0.5 had low sensitivities (54.6%, 47.9%, 21.9%, respectively), but were associated with relatively high specificities (73.7%, 81.7%, 95.7%, respectively) and negative predictive values (NPV) (99.2%, 99.2%, 99.0%, respectively), whereas positive predictive values (PPV) were low (2.5%, 3.2%, 6.0%, respectively). The authors concluded that due to the low sensitivity these CBC-derived indices do not represent reliable diagnostic markers to rule out EOS in neonates (Hornik et al., 2012). The very high negative predictive accuracy of more than 90% is in contrast to high rates of elevated IT-ratios between 25% and 50% in non-infected infants (Polin, 2012).

In a large historical cohort study comprising more than 3100 neonates, patients were evaluated for EOS. In this study a normal WBC was defined as an IT-ratio of less than 0.2 and a total WBC between 6000 and 30000/μL. Two serial normal WBCs with normal IT-ratios performed 8 to 12 hours apart and a negative blood culture at 24 hours were predictive of healthy newborns in the evaluation of EOS in the first 24 hours after birth and showed a negative predictive value of 100%. The sensitivity of 2 normal WBCs and a negative blood culture at 24 hours was 100%, as was NPV. The specificity was 51%, and the PPV was 8.8% (Murphy & Weiner, 2012). These results suggest that combinations of parameters and repeated performance of diagnostic tests are likely to increase accuracy.

In a review article Cornbleet reported a wide range of sensitivity and specificity for the IT-ratio and predicted a possible replacement by the measurement of newly created markers for infection such as inflammatory factors, adhesion molecules, cytokines, neutrophil surface antigens, and bacterial DNA (Cornbleet, 2002). Recent advances in basic science of predicting and diagnosing neonatal sepsis are developing towards more and more sophisticated approaches like the determination of proteomic inflammatory biomarkers in amniotic fluid (Buhimschi et al., 2009). Regarding these new techniques, the diagnostic value of traditional laboratory methods has to be critically analysed. However, comparing these new methods for the detection of neonatal sepsis with the measurement of WBCs including the assessment of the IG count (IGC) as well as the IT-ratio, the additional sample volumes, delayed availability of results, and considerably higher labour and laboratory costs should be taken into account.

1.1.2. Potential confounders in the manual assessment of IG by microscopic view of a manual smear

Anyhow, the detection of IGs by microscopic count necessitates experienced laboratory staff; furthermore morphological classification of IGs are subject to a considerable reader bias and interpretative errors; especially in neonates where leukocytosis occurs frequently in the first days of life this method seems to provide only limited reproducibility (Chiesa et al.,

2004; Schelonka et al., 1995). Contrariwise in performing a standard 100-cell manual differential small numbers of IGs are often underestimated as they can often be overlooked in samples of leukopenic patients. Another study highlighted the wide range of inter- and intraobserver variance in microscopic band cell identification: A smear of a blood sample from a septic patient was prepared, stained and a PowerPoint presentation was made twice of 100 random cells and sent to 157 different hospital laboratories in the Netherlands for a leukocyte differential. In the first survey neutrophils were differentiated in segmented and band neutrophils whereas in the second survey no discrimination was made between segmented and band neutrophils. Albeit the morphologic characteristics of a band cell are well defined, this study showed an enormous intervariability of enumeration of band cells so that the authors recommended to cease quantitative reporting of counted band cells especially in regard to other diagnostic tools like C-reactive protein (CRP), procalcitonin, and cytokines (van der Meer et al., 2006). Hence, several authors consider the manual count as inappropriate as a reference method for detection of IGs (Fernandes & Hamaguchi, 2007; Senthilnayagam et al., 2012).

2. Automated detection of immature granulocytes- Clinical applicability

Automated measurement of IGC could represent a reliable and utile method in the prediction of bacterial infection in neonates. In a study evaluating 106 samples from patients with an absolute neutrophil count (ANC) less than 2.0×10^9/L measured with an automated 5-part differential hematology instrument the IGC showed a very good precision and accuracy when compared with a flow cytometric neutrophil count using monoclonal antibodies for cell classification (Amundsen et al., 2012). In another investigation of 200 febrile patients suspected to have infection the performance characteristics of automated IGCs in predicting blood culture results and their clinical utility were assessed. The study population included adults, children, infants, and neonates. Measurements were performed using the Coulter Act Diff 5 counter which can perform a 5-part differential leucocyte count and can also numerate the percentage and absolute number of IG using a technology that combines cytochemistry, focused flow impedance, and light absorbance. The means of IGC and the percentage of IG (IG%) between culture positive and negative groups were statistically significant suggesting that they are potential markers for bacteremia. Among the 51 culture positive cases, 49 had an IT-ratio > 0.65% giving a sensitivity of 96.1%. IGC of $0.03 \times 10^3/\mu L$ and IG% of 0.5% offered a sensitivity of 86.3% and 92.2%, respectively. Higher values of IGC > 0.3 and IG% > 3 had a specificity greater than 90%, although the values were infrequent. Receiver operating characteristic (ROC) curves showed that IGC was a better predictor of infection than WBC and ANC in adults and the ratios IGC/WBC and IGC/ANC did not improve the prediction outcome (Senthilnayagam et al., 2012). Another study reported an in parallel increase of IG values to an increase of the ANC and an inverse relation to the lymphocyte count (Bernstein & Rucinski, 2011).

In an adult study population including patients suspected for sepsis higher percentages of IGs have been observed in infected than in non-infected patients and in patients with positive than patients with negative blood cultures (Ansari-Lari et al., 2003). Also in preterm hospitalized infants elevations of IGs were associated with positive blood culture results. In this study, values exceeding 0.5% showed a more than three-fold increased likelihood of a positive blood culture (Nigro et al., 2005).

In several studies comparing the manual microscopic method and the automated method for IG% and IGC significant correlation coefficients between 83% and 87% have been demonstrated (Field et al., 2006; Senthilnayagam et al., 2012). Compared with a flow cytometric reference count with monoclonal antibodies the correlation coefficient was even higher and amounted to 96% (Briggs et al., 2003). It has been shown that an increased percentage of more than 2% of IGs can be useful in identifying infection even when the neutrophil count is within the normal range and infection is not suspected. Conversely, in patients with a high IGC sample rates were positive for CRP and the erythrocyte sedimentation rate in 84% and 95%, respectively. Furthermore, elevated IGC showed a correlation with other inflammation markers such as CD 64 expression on polymorphonuclear cells and interleukin 6 concentration (Briggs et al., 2003).

The detection of IGs using automated hematology analyzers represents a fast, accurate, and less-labor intensive method and could improve screening and monitoring for neonatal septicaemia (Briggs et al., 2000; Fernandes & Hamaguchi, 2007; Nigro et al., 2005). The detection limit of IGs has been described to be 0.1% which is considerably lower than in a manual smear. The automated simultaneous enumeration of IGs in the course of performing a routine CBC provides additional information without the need of further costs and blood sampling, which might be of special importance in preterm babies. This new technology of automated measurement of IGs offers additional information reflecting the increase in bone marrow activity as an indicator of a left-shift of neutrophil cells in a more sensitive and specific way than the manual examination of a peripheral blood smear differential count.

Detection of IGs comprises the amount of metamyelocytes and myelocytes, but not band neutrophils and therefore reflects early stages of maturation of granulocytes. As the band cell is defined as a cell in the transitional state of granulopoetic maturation after the differentiation of metamyelocytes and myelocytes, the band count itself has been described as nonspecific, imprecise, and inaccurate as laboratory marker for the early detection of sepsis (Bernstein & Rucinski, 2011; Cornbleet, 2002). Hence, determination of IGs in contrast to the more mature band neutrophils, which arise later on, could be advantageous at the onset of moderate to severe inflammation (Cornbleet, 2002). Moreover, it has already been shown that the measurement of granulocyte maturation correlates to the identification of sepsis (Bernstein & Rucinski, 2011).

2.1. Neutrophil positional parameters as a new tool in the prediction of sepsis

Morphologic and physical properties of cells including cell volume, internal composition, and cytoplasmatic granularity and nuclear structure assessed via cell conductivity and cell scatter are described as positional parameters. In contrast to more mature cells IGs and band cells for instance are known to be larger, whereas nuclear composition is less complex. Based upon these facts positional parameters are used to classify different types of white blood cells, but recently this method has also been applied as a screening tool for neonatal sepsis to detect morphologic changes within the same blood cell population (i.e. in reactive neutrophil cells occurring during acute bacterial infection). Chaves et al. tried to assess and quantify these parameters as indicators of acute infection. In retrospective studies of adult septic patients and controls, the mean neutrophil volume (MNV) and its standard deviation, the neutrophil volume distribution width (NDW), reflecting the neutrophil size variability, showed high specifities (Chaves et al., 2005; 2006). In the control group the neutrophil population presented more homogenous than in bacteremic patients and the individual cell size varied less. Furthermore, a correlation of NDW respectively MNV and positive blood culture results, higher percentages of neutrophils and higher WBCs has been shown, whereas increased values were also present in patients without leukocytosis or neutrophilia possibly representing an important early diagnostic parameter in this subgroup of patients (Chaves et al., 2006). Another study using this technology showed good performance characteristics of MNV in detecting LOS in VLBW neonates with a NPV of 98.9%. Because of a considerably lower PPV the authors emphasize the possible combination with CRP-values in the prediction of sepsis. Interestingly, in contrast to an adult population the NDW did not reveal any clinical significance in a neonatal population. The authors suggested that this might be due to an originally more heterogeneous morphology of neutrophil cells in newborn infants (Raimondi et al., 2010; Raimondi et al., 2011).

2.2. The Sysmex XE-2100

The Sysmex XE-2100 (Sysmex Corporation, 2005), a multiparameter automated hematology analyzer offers the possibility to detect IGs including metamyelocytes, myelocytes, and promyelocytes by the measurement of white blood cell differential counts by flow cytometry in the DIFF-channel. Besides the quantification of IGs, physical properties of immature cells and reactivated neutrophils are provided. Therefore blood samples are incubated with Stromatolyser-IM, a fluorescent dye and a proprietary reagent, selectively leaking the membrane of mature leukocytes. Immature myeloid cells are not modified in their size, structure and integrity, because the IG has a lower cholesterol content than the mature granulocyte, and its phospholipid composition has a relatively higher ratio of phosphatidylcholine and a lower ratio of sphingomyelin (Gottfried, 1967). Depending on the dispersion angle when the cell passes the beam of a semiconductor laser, information about the volume, inner structure and complexity, and DNA/RNA content of each cell is obtained by a combination of forward-scattered light, lateral-scattered light, and lateral fluorescent light. The light is received by a photodiode respectively a photomultiplier tube and is then converted into electrical pulses. The higher content of RNA and DNA in IGs compared with segmented neutrophils is reflected in an increased fluorescence emission after excitation with the laser beam. The XE-2100 is equipped with an additional immature information (IMI) channel, where not only IGs, but also bands, blasts, and hematopoietic progenitor cells are detected. Detection of cell size, information about the nuclei and composition of cytoplasm is generated by direct current and radio frequency resistance when cells pass an aperture in the IMI-channel. The direct current (DC) pulse height is equivalent to cell volume. The radio frequency (RF) measurement provides information on the internal composition of the cell (nucleus, granules). Differences in RF resistance detected as electrical pulses are plotted in a two dimensional scattergram reflecting the distribution of cell and nucleus size (Sysmex Corporation, 2005).

The IMI-channel determines the total number of myeloid precursor cells by distinguishing selectively immature myeloid cells from mature leukocytes. The reaction principle of the IMI-channel is based on differences in membrane composition between mature and immature cells. It has been shown that the flow cytometric IGC performed by the Sysmex XE-2100 is superior to the manual morphology count as a reference method for IG counting and that the percentage of IGs is a better predictor of infection than the WBC (Ansari-Lari et al., 2003; Fernandes & Hamaguchi, 2007).

3. Reference values in an adult and pediatric population

Generally, normal values of laboratory parameters in a neonatal population are difficult to define, because removal of blood is usually not performed in healthy neonates and reference ranges are composed by assessing patients with minor illness (Christensen et al., 2009). To our knowledge, the first published reference values for neutrophil cells in neonates including the total neutrophil count, the absolute number of immature neutrophils, and the IT-ratio during the first 28 days of life refers to a study by Manroe in 1979 (Manroe et al., 1979). About 15 years later the same study group found that in VLBW these reference values are of limited applicability because a wider range of distribution was found in this subgroup of patients compared to larger or older counterparts (Mouzinho et al., 1994). These new data comprised a wider range of the absolute total neutrophil count and a considerable decreased lower limit in the first 60 hours after birth, whereas reference ranges for the immature neutrophil count and IT values remain unchanged. It has been assumed that low neutrophil counts soon after birth might be caused by a placental factor inhibiting neutrophil production. Clearance of this factor within the first week could lead to the observed increase in immature neutrophil cells. Anyhow, the capability of the bone marrow to rapidly produce immature as well as mature neutrophil forms by the second week is well documented. Neutropenia occurred rarely in infants at an age of more than 7 days, but neutrophilia occurred frequently in association with stress conditions inducing an adrenergic increase in cyclic adenosine monophosphate (cAMP) leading to a release of neutrophil cells (Mouzinho et al., 1994). Hence, neutropenia has been described as a better predictor for neonatal sepsis than an elevated neutrophil count because besides accelerated utilization in case of infection there a fewer factors (i.e. hemolytic disease, asphyxia, maternal hypertension) causing a decrease of neutrophil granulocytes. Lower levels of normal for neutrophil values have been set at 1800/mm^3 at birth and < 7800/mm^3 12-14 hours after birth in term and late preterm infants (Manroe et al., 1979).

A large trial evaluating more than 30000 samples from infants born at 23 to 42 weeks of gestational age reinvestigated the previously published reference ranges using an automated blood cell counter (Schmutz et al., 2008). In this study lower limits of normal for the neutrophil count were determined as follows (Table 1):

Gestational age	Neutrophil count at birth	Neutrophil count 6-8h pn
> 36 weeks	3500/μL	7500/μL
28-36 weeks	1000/μL	3500/μL
< 28 weeks	500/μL	1500/μL

Table 1. Neutrophil count at birth and 6-8 hours postnatally (pn) comparing groups of different gestational age (Polin, 2012; Schmutz et al., 2008).

The notable difference in altitude between the two studies might have influenced the results. The dynamic process of granulopoesis after birth is reflected by a rapid increase of neutrophil cells reaching peak levels at 6 to 8 hours postnatally (Polin, 2012; Schmutz et al., 2008). Allowing sufficient reaction time to inflammatory stimuli alterations in mature and immature granulocytes are more likely to occur between 6 to 12 hours after birth. This should be taken into account when planning blood sampling (Polin, 2012).

A quite similar time course has been shown for the absolute immature neutrophil count: Maximal values increase from 1100/μL soon after birth to a peak of 1500/μL at 12 hours postnatally. In contrast to that, maximum normal values for the IT-ratio have been observed directly after birth followed by a decline with increasing age (Polin, 2012; Schmutz et al., 2008). In the most immature infants between 24 and 26 weeks of gestational age, an elevation of ANC has been shown during the first month of life. In the first three weeks of life a weekly decrease of ANC to values between 2000/μL and 4000/μL has been observed. As the prevalence of both neutropenia as well as neutrophilia decreased with maturity, it can be concluded that granulopoetic function stabilizes with higher gestational age enabling adequate reactions to infectious or stress stimuli. Deviations from the normal range of neutrophil granulocytes without additional signs of clinical symptoms or conditions occurred frequently even in a hospitalized population (Juul et al., 2004). In the face of these data more interest should be attracted on considering the gestational age as well as the time point of blood sampling when interpreting CBC results (Polin, 2012). The influence of birth weight on CBC in healthy term infants was examined in a study performed by Ozyürek and co-workers. Their data revealed a clear difference in several CBC parameters comparing healthy, term infants with intrauterine growth retardation to appropriate for gestational age (AGA) counterparts showing neutropenia in 21% as well as higher IT-ratios in small for gestational age (SGA) newborns. Beyond these findings, a higher rate in immature neutrophil cells, namely in the absolute number of metamyeolcytes, was observed in the SGA babies. The authors suggested that this elevation might be interpreted as a reaction of the bone marrow to compensate for the initially frequent low neutrophil count (Ozyurek et al., 2006).

Some authors have considered the method of automated measurement of IGC as not sensitive enough to be used as a sole screening assay for the prediction of infection. However, it has been demonstrated that a high percentage of IG (> 3%) is a very specific predictor (> 90%) of sepsis (Ansari-Lari et al., 2003) and that IG values less than 0.5% are associated with a high negative predictive value. These findings might be of use in a clinical context (Nigro et al., 2005). Recently published reference values have defined a median of $0.63 x 10^3$/μL (0.1–2.4; 2.5%–97.5% confidence interval) for IG number (IG#) and a cut-off value of 3.2% for IG% as optimal for a normal adult population. Using a cut-off in a range between 4% and 5% of total WBC would result in a too high rate of missed cases (Bernstein & Rucinski, 2011). In a large outpatient pediatric population comprising more than 2400 samples, age dependent upper limits for reference ranges for the automated enumeration of IG were defined as 0.30% and 40/μL for IG% and IG#, respectively for children aged below 10 years (Roehrl et al., 2011). Above the age of 10 years, an upper limit of 0.90% and 70.0/μL for relative and absolute IG count was recommended (Roehrl et al., 2011). In this study blood samples were analyzed using the Sysmex XT-1800i instrument (Sysmex, Kobe, Japan). The defined upper limits showed no differences dependent on the patient sex. As expected the cause of elevated IGC differed between both groups. While respiratory or gastrointestinal infections were common associations with elevated IGC in the group < 10 years, the older children showed hematologic malignancies, drug therapy (glucocorticoids, chemotherapy), severe infections, and pregnancy (young females). In a subgroup analysis of patients < 1 year this study revealed age-stratified nonparametric estimates of upper limits of normal (95th percentiles) and associated 90% confidence intervals (CI) for IG# and IG% of 40/μL (30.0–50.0) and 0.30% (0.20–0.40). In addition, this study described an important observation: Even the most abnormal IGCs in the younger age group were quite low compared with abnormal IGCs in the older individuals. This fact highlights the importance of particular reference values appropriate for different age groups. Otherwise especially younger children with associated disease and with only small elevations of IGCs could be overlooked (Roehrl et al., 2011). As neonates represent a highly particular and often vulnerable patient population we aimed at investigate a possible correlation between IGC and sepsis.

3.1. "The predictive value of immature granulocyte count and immature myeloid information in the diagnosis of neonatal sepsis"- own experience and study results

Our study group tried to determine the predictive value of the IG# and the immature myeloid information (IMI) in neonatal early onset sepsis performing a historical cohort study (Cimenti et al., 2012).

3.1.1. Patients and methods

We collected 133 blood samples of neonates admitted to the NICU of the Pediatric Department of the Medical University Graz, a tertiary care center. Based on their admission diagnosis and their clinical course patients were divided in two groups. The first group consisted of patients with blood culture verified bacteremia, clinically strongly suspected sepsis, or elevated inflammatory parameters, a history of risk factors, and antibiotic treatment ≥ 7 d. Patients in the second group were asymptomatic, healthy children without any infectious risk factors constituting the control group. They were admitted to the NICU because of low birth weight, delayed postnatal transition or prematurity.

Blood sampling was routinely performed in all neonates and repeated depending on their clinical course. Blood samples were collected into microvette tubes (Sarstedt, Nümbrecht, Germany) and analyzed using the Sysmex XE-2100 (13). In cases of suspected bacterial infection, blood samples were always taken before the initiation of antibiotic therapy. ROC curves were used for comparison of infectious indices by plotting the test sensitivity (equivalent to the true positive rate) on the y-axis and 1-specifity (equivalent to the false positive rate) on the x-axis for all possible cut off values of the diagnostic test (see Figure 1).

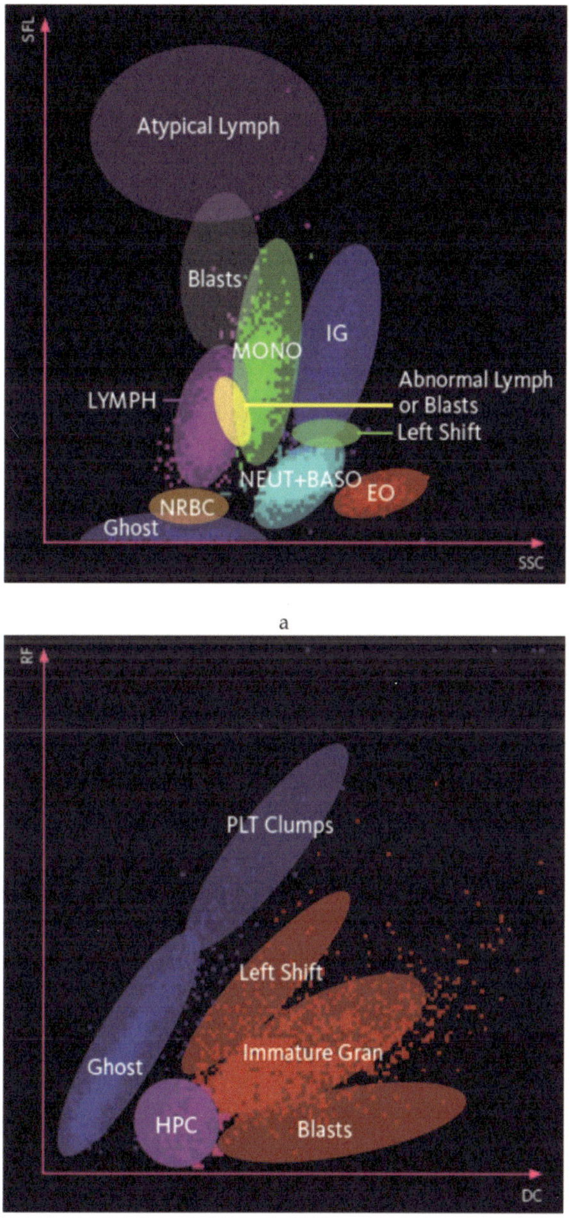

a

b

Figure 1. a and b: Diff- and IMI scattergram showing graphic output of WBC differential results performed with the Sysmex XE 2100. By courtesy of © Sysmex Europe GmbH, Norderstedt, Germany.

The Youden's index (sensitivity in %)/100 + (specificity in % - 1)/100 - 1 was used for determination of optimal cut-off values. The area under the curve (AUC) was calculated using the binormal approach by McClish. ROC curve are used to assess the diagnostic accuracy of a test. The ROC curve allows analyses of the trade-offs between sensitivity and specificity at all possible cut-off points and is often used to determine optimal cut-off values and to compare the usefulness of two more diagnostic tests. The area under the curve (AUC) is another useful tool describing the discriminative ability of a test across the full range of cut-offs. A test with an AUC greater than 0.9 has high accuracy, while 0.7–0.9 describes moderate accuracy, 0.5–0.7 implies low accuracy and 0.5 displays a chance result (Akobeng, 2007; Fischer et al., 2003).

Of 133 blood samples of patients admitted to our neonatal intensive care unit 21 neonates were suspected and treated for sepsis (mean gestational age 34.1 weeks, mean birth weight 2287 g, 9 male, 12 female, 12 patients had a history of premature rupture of membranes (PROM)). In the control group 112 healthy neonates were analyzed (mean gestational age 34.2 weeks, mean birth weight 2128 g, 59 male, 53 female, 31 patients with a history of PROM).

3.1.2. Results

The number of IMI classified cells (IMI#) was significantly elevated in patients with sepsis compared to the control group (639/μL (144; 2029) vs. 89/μL (40; 133), p=0.000065). The number of IMI/ total leucocyte count (IMI%) in patients with sepsis was significantly elevated compared to the control group (4.5 (1.3; 9.5) vs. 0.7 (0.5; 1.1), values expressed in %, p=0.000076). IG# was significantly elevated in neonates with sepsis compared to the control group (0.28x 10^3/μL (0.03; 0.56) vs. 0.05x10^3/μL (0.05-0.09), p=0.049). The percentage of IG% was significantly elevated in septic neonates vs. infants in the control group (1.3 (0.5; 4.5) vs. 0.5 (0.4; 0.7), values expressed in %, p=0.022) (Cimenti et al., 2012). The AUC for the IMI# was 0.76 and 0.70 for IG% and IMI%, respectively. The positive and negative predictive value, sensitivity, specificity, and the Youden's index at different cut off values are listed in Table 2 (Cimenti et al., 2012).

Parameter	Cut-off	PPV	NPV	sensitivity	specificity	Youden'sindex
IG#	0.24	0.60	0.31	0.60	0.88	0.48
IG%	1.3	0.67	0.27	0.67	0.88	0.55
IMI#	262	0.80	0.09	0.80	0.72	0.52
IMI%	0.02	0.70	0.14	0.70	0.76	0.46
IT ratio	0.06	0.75	0.20	0.75	0.94	0.69

Table 2. Positive predictive value, negative predictive value, sensitivity, and specificity of IG#, IG%, IMI#, IMI% and IT ratio for optimal cut off values determined by ROC analysis using the Youden's index in 21 neonates with sepsis compared to 112 neonates with negative infectious status (Cimenti et al., 2012).

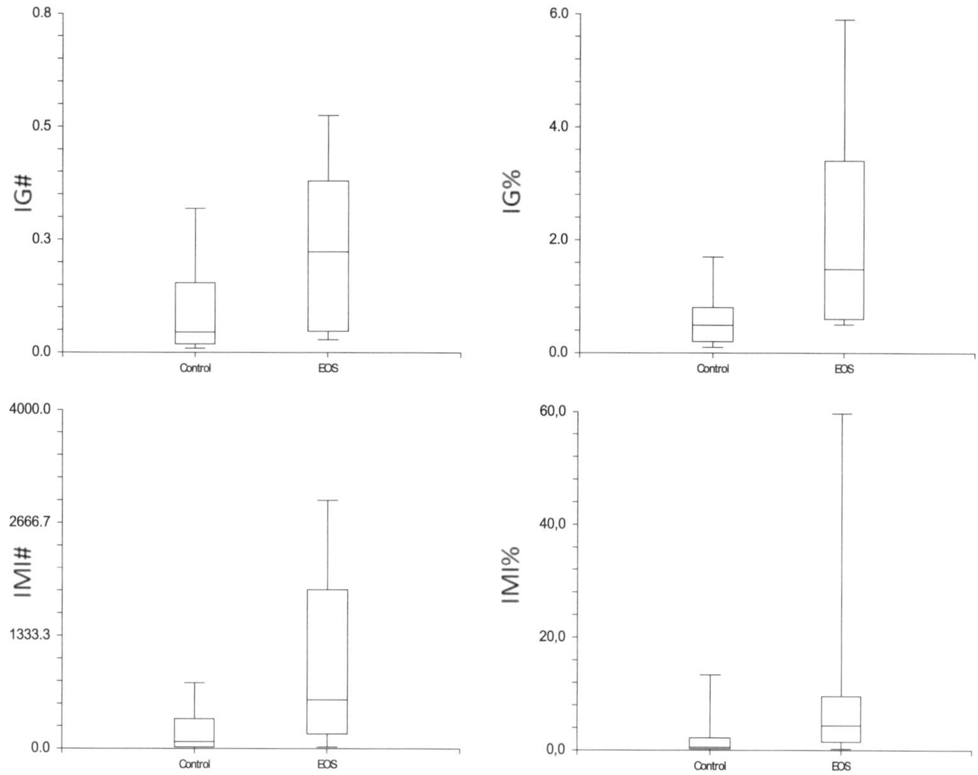

Figure 2. Boxplot diagram showing the distribution of IG#, IG%, IMI#, and IMI% values in neonates with sepsis compared to the control group. The top and the bottom of the box represent the 25th and 75th percentile; the line in the box indicates the median. The whiskers display the largest data less than or equal to the 75th percentile plus 1.5 times interquartile range and the lowest data greater than or equal to the 25th percentile minus 1.5 times interquartile range (Cimenti et al., 2012).

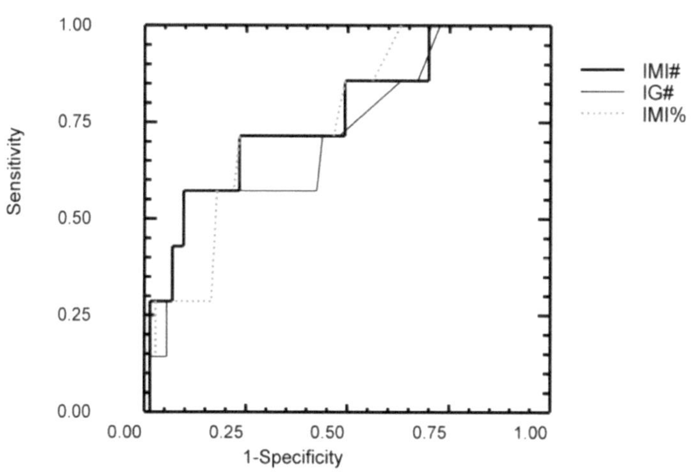

Figure 3. Receiver operating characteristic (ROC) curves of IMI# (thick line), IG# (thin line) and IMI% (dotted line).

3.1.3. Reference values for a neonatal study population based on ROC analysis

Preliminary data revealed a cut-off value for IG% of 1.3% based on calculations using the Youden's index and a median of $0.05 \times 10^3/\mu L$ (0.05-0.09; 2.5%–97.5% confidence interval) for IG# in our control group of asymptomatic, healthy subjects. According to our data the measurement of IMI# compared to IG# seems to be more favourable as determined by ROC analysis as there seems to be a tendency that the IM# has a higher predictive value than the IG# (Figure 3). Setting a cut off value of 262/μl the measurement of IMI# revealed a positive predictive value of 0.80.

3.2. Possible limitations of the use of IG

White blood cell differential counts are not only influenced by infection. The gestational as well as the infant's age in hours at the time of blood collection, the method of blood sampling and the infant's gender might affect the results as well as the method of delivery, or maternal risk factors like hypertension (Chirico et al., 1999; Christensen et al., 2009; Escobar, 2003; Kayiran et al., 2003; Newman et al., 2010; Schelonka et al., 1995; Schmutz et al., 2008). Even the influence of the sea level on ANC in neonates has been described leading to a wider range of reference values with isolated elevated counts of absolute neutrophil granulocytes but normal IT-ratios in healthy term babies (Lambert et al., 2009).

A prospective longitudinal study observed higher cord blood cortisol levels, as a sensitive marker of intrauterine stress, in infants born by vaginal delivery compared to elective cesarean section in term neonates and a significant positive correlation between total leukocyte and neutrophil counts. After 12 hours of life no differences in the variation of leukocyte counts remained. Although a significant increase of immature neutrophil counts in vaginally delivered infants or after long labour has been previously described (Hasan et al., 1993; Schelonka et al., 1994), no significant differences in the IT-ratio were detected between the two groups (Chirico et al., 1999). In a prospective observational study including 60 preterm infants with a gestational age < 32 weeks prenatal growth retardation has been shown to be an independent factor for significantly lower counts of leukocytes, total neutrophil and immature neutrophil counts in very immature preterm infants immediately after birth when compared with AGA counterparts. It has been assumed that these low numbers of circulating white blood cells might reflect the reduced bone marrow reserves (Wirbelauer et al., 2010). As the median granulocyte count in the SGA group was with a count of 1.058/μL near to absolute granulopenia one could consider this as a risk factor for sepsis, as previous studies had reported an association between early onset neutropenia and sepsis (Christensen et al., 2006). But low numbers of inflammatory cells could also represent a possible protection mechanism for pulmonary and central-nervous disease by reducing inflammatory events postnatally (Wirbelauer et al., 2010). Among extremely low birth weight (ELBW) neonates low neutrophil counts (< 1000/μL) have been observed with a rate of five times higher than reported in the general NICU population. Most cases were present in the first days of life and represented a transient phenomenon. SGA or maternal pregnancy induced hypertension were common causes for these alterations, whereas in over one third of cases no cause had been detected. Except in proven early onset bacterial infection, the presence, severity and duration of low counts showed no relationship with mortality rate, whereas neutropenia within the first 3 days of life showed an association with necrotizing enterocolitis (NEC) or nosocomial infection (Christensen et al., 2006).Using IGC in a clinical context should incorporate these factors as well as the likelihood of infection in every individual patient.

As for the blood cell count it has been shown that the performance characteristics in distinguishing between infants with and without infections improve significantly during the first 4 hours after birth. The AUC of the WBC, ANC and IT-ratio showed an increase from 0 hours of 0.52, 0.55 and 0.73, respectively to 0.87, 0.85 and 0.82, respectively 4 hours after birth (Newman et al., 2010). In a review article on new technologies for a diagnostic approach in neonatal sepsis Srinivasan and Harris considered the future development of computerized algorithms including these variables as possibly useful to estimate the probability of sepsis (Srinivasan & Harris, 2012). Taking this fact into account it might be advisable to perform serial IGCs, especially in cases where sepsis had to be ruled out and the result of the test will have a therapeutic consequence (i.e. discontinuing of antibiotic treatment).

The clinical applicability of automated IG counting might be limited by the relatively poor sensitivity of this method (Ansari-Lari et al., 2003; Nigro et al., 2005). Considering the satisfactory specificity and the high NPV this parameter could represent a valuable additional aid in combination with other laboratory markers or diagnostic algorithms. However, as higher values of IG% of more than 3% have been shown to predict blood culture positive results (Ansari-Lari et al., 2003), this subgroup of patients should probably be revaluated for potential infection even in the absence of specific symptoms.

4. Conclusion

As clinical signs in preterm and term infants with severe bacterial infection are often non-specific and scarce, automated detection of IGs and IMI seems to act as a useful adjunctive tool in the diagnosis of neonatal sepsis. Technical development of automated hematology analyzers has led to a precise, fast, accurate, and reproducible determination of IGs. The detection of all immature cells including blasts in a separate channel might be advantageous at an early stage of sepsis, when these cells are released from bone marrow and the peripheral neutrophil count can still be in the normal range.

Although automated determination of IGs is currently carried out in the area of research, evidence exists that this method seems to be worth to be implemented in clinical practice especially as an adjunctive tool in determining early phase of bacterial sepsis. The fact that measurement of this parameter in the course of routine determination of a white blood differential count does not necessitate any additional sample volume, personal effort, or costs, might be a valuable additional argument. Further well designed prospective trials are mandatory to validate the performance characteristics of these new parameters as diagnostic tool in neonatal sepsis. In this context, the availability of an internal quality control and the development and implementation of external quality assessment schemes to evaluate analytical performance, compare different laboratories and methods as well as the definition of standards represent indispensable conditions for a reasonable use in clinical routine (Briggs, 2009).

Author details

Christina Cimenti, Wolfgang Erwa, Wilhelm Müller, Bernhard Resch
Medical University Graz, Austria

5. References

Akenzua, G.I., Hui, Y.T., Milner, R., & Zipursky, A. (1974). Neutrophil and band counts in the diagnosis of neonatal infections. Pediatrics, Vol.54, No.1 (Jul, 1974), pp. (38-42), ISSN 0031-4005.

Akobeng, A.K. (2007). Understanding diagnostic tests 3: Receiver operating characteristic curves. Acta Paediatr, Vol.96, No.5 (May, 2007), pp. (644-7), ISSN 0803-5253.

Amundsen, E.K., Urdal, P., Hagve, T.A., Holthe, M.R., & Henriksson, C.E. (2012). Absolute neutrophil counts from automated hematology instruments are accurate and precise even at very low levels. Am J Clin Pathol, Vol.137, No.6 (Jun, 2012), pp. (862-9), ISSN 1943-7722.

Ansari-Lari, M.A., Kickler, T.S., & Borowitz, M.J. (2003). Immature Granulocyte Measurement Using the Sysmex XE-2100 Relationship to Infection and Sepsis. American Journal of Clinical Pathology, Vol.120, No.5 (2003), pp. (795-9), ISSN 0002-9173.

Azizia, M., Lloyd, J., Allen, M., Klein, N., & Peebles, D. (2012). Immune status in very preterm neonates. Pediatrics, Vol.129, No.4 (Apr, 2012), pp. (e967-74), ISSN 1098-4275.

Bernstein, L.H., & Rucinski, J. (2011). Measurement of granulocyte maturation may improve the early diagnosis of the septic state. Clin Chem Lab Med, (Sep 21, 2011), pp., ISSN 1434-6621.

Briggs, C., Harrison, P., Grant, D., Staves, J., & MacHin, S.J. (2000). New quantitative parameters on a recently introduced automated blood cell counter--the XE 2100. Clin Lab Haematol, Vol.22, No.6 (Dec, 2000), pp. (345-50), ISSN 0141-9854.

Briggs, C., Kunka, S., Fujimoto, H., Hamaguchi, Y., Davis, B.H., & Machin, S.J. (2003). Evaluation of immature granulocyte counts by the XE-IG master: upgraded software for the XE-2100 automated hematology analyzer. Lab Hematol, Vol.9, No.3 (2003), pp. (117-24), ISSN 1080-2924.

Briggs, C. (2009). Quality counts: new parameters in blood cell counting. Int J Lab Hematol, Vol.31, No.3 (Jun, 2009), pp. (277-97), ISSN 1751-553X.

Buhimschi, C.S., Bhandari, V., Han, Y.W., Dulay, A.T., Baumbusch, M.A., Madri, J.A., & Buhimschi, I.A. (2009). Using proteomics in perinatal and neonatal sepsis: hopes and challenges for the future. Curr Opin Infect Dis, Vol.22, No.3 (Jun, 2009), pp. (235-43), ISSN 1473-6527.

Buttarello, M., & Plebani, M. (2008). Automated blood cell counts: state of the art. Am J Clin Pathol, Vol.130, No.1 (Jul, 2008), pp. (104-16), ISSN 0002-9173.

Chaves, F., Tierno, B., & Xu, D. (2005). Quantitative determination of neutrophil VCS parameters by the Coulter automated hematology analyzer: new and reliable indicators for acute bacterial infection. Am J Clin Pathol, Vol.124, No.3 (Sep, 2005), pp. (440-4), ISSN 0002-9173.

Chaves, F., Tierno, B., & Xu, D. (2006). Neutrophil volume distribution width: a new automated hematologic parameter for acute infection. Arch Pathol Lab Med, Vol.130, No.3 (Mar, 2006), pp. (378-80), ISSN 1543-2165.

Chiesa, C., Panero, A., Osborn, J.F., Simonetti, A.F., & Pacifico, L. (2004). Diagnosis of neonatal sepsis: a clinical and laboratory challenge. Clin Chem, Vol.50, No.2 (Feb, 2004), pp. (279-87), ISSN 0009-9147.

Chirico, G., Gasparoni, A., Ciardelli, L., Martinotti, L., & Rondini, G. (1999). Leukocyte counts in relation to the method of delivery during the first five days of life. Biol Neonate, Vol.75, No.5 (May, 1999), pp. (294-9), ISSN 0006-3126.

Christensen, R.D., Bradley, P.P., & Rothstein, G. (1981). The leukocyte left shift in clinical and experimental neonatal sepsis. J Pediatr, Vol.98, No.1 (Jan, 1981), pp. (101-5), ISSN 0022-3476.

Christensen, R.D., Henry, E., Wiedmeier, S.E., Stoddard, R.A., & Lambert, D.K. (2006). Low blood neutrophil concentrations among extremely low birth weight neonates: data from a multihospital health-care system. J Perinatol, Vol.26, No.11 (Nov, 2006), pp. (682-7), ISSN 0743-8346.

Christensen, R.D., Henry, E., Jopling, J., & Wiedmeier, S.E. (2009). The CBC: reference ranges for neonates. Semin Perinatol, Vol.33, No.1 (Feb, 2009), pp. (3-11), ISSN 1558-075X.

Cimenti, C., Erwa, W., Herkner, K.R., Kasper, D.C., Muller, W., & Resch, B. (2012). The predictive value of immature granulocyte count and immature myeloid information in the diagnosis of neonatal sepsis. Clin Chem Lab Med, Vol.50, No.8 (2012), pp. (1429-32), ISSN 1434-6621.

Cornbleet, P.J. (2002). Clinical utility of the band count. Clin Lab Med, Vol.22, No.1 (Mar, 2002), pp. (101-36), ISSN 0272-2712.

Escobar, G.J. (2003). Effect of the systemic inflammatory response on biochemical markers of neonatal bacterial infection: a fresh look at old confounders. Clin Chem, Vol.49, No.1 (Jan, 2003), pp. (21-2), ISSN 0009-9147.

Fanaroff, A.A., Stoll, B.J., Wright, L.L., Carlo, W.A., Ehrenkranz, R.A., Stark, A.R., Bauer, C.R., Donovan, E.F., Korones, S.B., Laptook, A.R., Lemons, J.A., Oh, W., Papile, L.A., Shankaran, S., Stevenson, D.K., Tyson, J.E., & Poole, W.K. (2007). Trends in neonatal morbidity and mortality for very low birthweight infants. Am J Obstet Gynecol, Vol.196, No.2 (Feb, 2007), pp. (147 e1-8), ISSN 1097-6868.

Fernandes, B., & Hamaguchi, Y. (2007). Automated Enumeration of Immature Granulocytes. American Journal of Clinical Pathology, Vol.128, No.3 (2007), pp. (454-63), ISSN 0002-9173.

Field, D., Taube, E., & Heumann, S. (2006). Performance evaluation of the immature granulocyte parameter on the Sysmex XE-2100 automated hematology analyzer. Lab Hematol, Vol.12, No.1 (2006), pp. (11-4), ISSN 1080-2924.

Fischer, J.E., Bachmann, L.M., & Jaeschke, R. (2003). A readers' guide to the interpretation of diagnostic test properties: clinical example of sepsis. Intensive Care Med, Vol.29, No.7 (Jul, 2003), pp. (1043-51), ISSN 0342-4642.

Fowlie, P.W., & Schmidt, B. (1998). Diagnostic tests for bacterial infection from birth to 90 days--a systematic review. Arch Dis Child Fetal Neonatal Ed, Vol.78, No.2 (Mar, 1998), pp. (F92-8), ISSN 1359-2998.

Gottfried, E.L. (1967). Lipids of human leukocytes: relation to celltype. J Lipid Res, Vol.8, No.4 (Jul, 1967), pp. (321-7), ISSN 0022-2275.

Guerti, K., Devos, H., Ieven, M.M., & Mahieu, L.M. (2011). Time to positivity of neonatal blood cultures: fast and furious? J Med Microbiol, Vol.60, No.Pt 4 (Apr, 2011), pp. (446-53), ISSN 1473-5644.

Haque, K.N. (2010). Neonatal Sepsis in the Very Low Birth Weight Preterm Infants: Part 2: Review of Definition, Diagnosis and Management. Journal of Medical Sciences, Vol.3, No.1 (2010), pp. (11-27).

Hasan, R., Inoue, S., & Banerjee, A. (1993). Higher white blood cell counts and band forms in newborns delivered vaginally compared with those delivered by cesarean section. Am J Clin Pathol, Vol.100, No.2 (Aug, 1993), pp. (116-8), ISSN 0002-9173.

Hornik, C.P., Benjamin, D.K., Becker, K.C., Benjamin, D.K., Jr., Li, J., Clark, R.H., Cohen-Wolkowiez, M., & Smith, P.B. (2012). Use of the Complete Blood Cell Count in Early-Onset Neonatal Sepsis. Pediatr Infect Dis J, (Apr 23, 2012), pp., ISSN 1532-0987.

Juul, S.E., Haynes, J.W., & McPherson, R.J. (2004). Evaluation of neutropenia and neutrophilia in hospitalized preterm infants. J Perinatol, Vol.24, No.3 (Mar, 2004), pp. (150-7), ISSN 0743-8346.

Kayiran, S.M., Ozbek, N., Turan, M., & Gurakan, B. (2003). Significant differences between capillary and venous complete blood counts in the neonatal period. Clin Lab Haematol, Vol.25, No.1 (Feb, 2003), pp. (9-16), ISSN 0141-9854.

Kellogg, J.A., Ferrentino, F.L., Goodstein, M.H., Liss, J., Shapiro, S.L., & Bankert, D.A. (1997). Frequency of low level bacteremia in infants from birth to two months of age. Pediatr Infect Dis J, Vol.16, No.4 (Apr, 1997), pp. (381-5), ISSN 0891-3668.

Lambert, R.M., Baer, V.L., Wiedmeier, S.E., Henry, E., Burnett, J., & Christensen, R.D. (2009). Isolated elevated blood neutrophil concentration at altitude does not require NICU admission if appropriate reference ranges are used. J Perinatol, Vol.29, No.12 (Dec, 2009), pp. (822-5), ISSN 1476-5543.

Manroe, B.L., Weinberg, A.G., Rosenfeld, C.R., & Browne, R. (1979). The neonatal blood count in health and disease. I. Reference values for neutrophilic cells. J Pediatr, Vol.95, No.1 (Jul, 1979), pp. (89-98), ISSN 0022-3476.

Mouzinho, A., Rosenfeld, C.R., Sanchez, P.J., & Risser, R. (1994). Revised reference ranges for circulating neutrophils in very-low-birth-weight neonates. Pediatrics, Vol.94, No.1 (Jul, 1994), pp. (76-82), ISSN 0031-4005.

Murphy, K., & Weiner, J. (2012). Use of leukocyte counts in evaluation of early-onset neonatal sepsis. Pediatr Infect Dis J, Vol.31, No.1 (Jan, 2012), pp. (16-9), ISSN 1532-0987.

Newman, T.B., Puopolo, K.M., Wi, S., Draper, D., & Escobar, G.J. (2010). Interpreting complete blood counts soon after birth in newborns at risk for sepsis. Pediatrics, Vol.126, No.5 (Nov, 2010), pp. (903-9), ISSN 1098-4275.

Nigro, K.G., O'Riordan, M., Molloy, E.J., Walsh, M.C., & Sandhaus, L.M. (2005). Performance of an automated immature granulocyte count as a predictor of neonatal sepsis. Am J Clin Pathol, Vol.123, No.4 (Apr, 2005), pp. (618-24), ISSN 0002-9173.

Ottolini, M.C., Lundgren, K., Mirkinson, L.J., Cason, S., & Ottolini, M.G. (2003). Utility of complete blood count and blood culture screening to diagnose neonatal sepsis in the asymptomatic at risk newborn. Pediatr Infect Dis J, Vol.22, No.5 (May, 2003), pp. (430-4), ISSN 0891-3668.

Ozyurek, E., Cetintas, S., Ceylan, T., Ogus, E., Haberal, A., Gurakan, B., & Ozbek, N. (2006). Complete blood count parameters for healthy, small-for-gestational-age, full-term newborns. Clin Lab Haematol, Vol.28, No.2 (Apr, 2006), pp. (97-104), ISSN 0141-9854.

Polin, R.A. (2012). Management of neonates with suspected or proven early-onset bacterial sepsis. Pediatrics, Vol.129, No.5 (May, 2012), pp. (1006-15), ISSN 1098-4275.

Pourcyrous, M., Bada, H.S., Korones, S.B., Baselski, V., & Wong, S.P. (1993). Significance of serial C-reactive protein responses in neonatal infection and other disorders. Pediatrics, Vol.92, No.3 (Sep, 1993), pp. (431-5), ISSN 0031-4005.

Raimondi, F., Ferrara, T., Capasso, L., Sellitto, M., Landolfo, F., Romano, A., Grimaldi, E., & Scopacasa, F. (2010). Automated determination of neutrophil volume as screening test for late-onset sepsis in very low birth infants. Pediatr Infect Dis J, Vol.29, No.3 (Mar, 2010), pp. (288), ISSN 1532-0987.

Raimondi, F., Ferrara, T., Maffucci, R., Milite, P., Del Buono, D., Santoro, P., & Grimaldi, L.C. (2011). Neonatal sepsis: a difficult diagnostic challenge. Clin Biochem, Vol.44, No.7 (May, 2011), pp. (463-4), ISSN 1873-2933.

Rodwell, R.L., Leslie, A.L., & Tudehope, D.I. (1988). Early diagnosis of neonatal sepsis using a hematologic scoring system. J Pediatr, Vol.112, No.5 (May, 1988), pp. (761-7), ISSN 0022-3476.

Roehrl, M.H., Lantz, D., Sylvester, C., & Wang, J.Y. (2011). Age-dependent reference ranges for automated assessment of immature granulocytes and clinical significance in an outpatient setting. Arch Pathol Lab Med, Vol.135, No.4 (Apr, 2011), pp. (471-7), ISSN 1543-2165.

Rozycki, H.J., Stahl, G.E., & Baumgart, S. (1987). Impaired sensitivity of a single early leukocyte count in screening for neonatal sepsis. Pediatr Infect Dis J, Vol.6, No.5 (May, 1987), pp. (440-2), ISSN 0891-3668.

Schelonka, R.L., Yoder, B.A., desJardins, S.E., Hall, R.B., & Butler, J. (1994). Peripheral leukocyte count and leukocyte indexes in healthy newborn term infants. J Pediatr, Vol.125, No.4 (Oct, 1994), pp. (603-6), ISSN 0022-3476.

Schelonka, R.L., Yoder, B.A., Hall, R.B., Trippett, T.M., Louder, D.S., Hickman, J.R., & Guerra, C.G. (1995). Differentiation of segmented and band neutrophils during the early newborn period. J Pediatr, Vol.127, No.2 (Aug, 1995), pp. (298-300), ISSN 0022-3476.

Schelonka, R.L., Chai, M.K., Yoder, B.A., Hensley, D., Brockett, R.M., & Ascher, D.P. (1996). Volume of blood required to detect common neonatal pathogens. J Pediatr, Vol.129, No.2 (Aug, 1996), pp. (275-8), ISSN 0022-3476.

Schmutz, N., Henry, E., Jopling, J., & Christensen, R.D. (2008). Expected ranges for blood neutrophil concentrations of neonates: the Manroe and Mouzinho charts revisited. J Perinatol, Vol.28, No.4 (Apr, 2008), pp. (275-81), ISSN 0743-8346.

Senthilnayagam, B., Kumar, T., Sukumaran, J., M, J., & Rao, K.R. (2012). Automated measurement of immature granulocytes: performance characteristics and utility in routine clinical practice. Patholog Res Int, Vol.2012, (2012), pp. (483670), ISSN 2042-003X.

Srinivasan, L., & Harris, M.C. (2012). New technologies for the rapid diagnosis of neonatal sepsis. Curr Opin Pediatr, Vol.24, No.2 (Apr, 2012), pp. (165-71), ISSN 1531-698X.

Stoll, B.J., Gordon, T., Korones, S.B., Shankaran, S., Tyson, J.E., Bauer, C.R., Fanaroff, A.A., Lemons, J.A., Donovan, E.F., Oh, W., Stevenson, D.K., Ehrenkranz, R.A., Papile, L.A., Verter, J., & Wright, L.L. (1996). Early-onset sepsis in very low birth weight neonates: a report from the National Institute of Child Health and Human Development Neonatal Research Network. J Pediatr, Vol.129, No.1 (Jul, 1996), pp. (72-80), ISSN 0022-3476.

Stoll, B.J., Hansen, N.I., Adams-Chapman, I., Fanaroff, A.A., Hintz, S.R., Vohr, B., & Higgins, R.D. (2004). Neurodevelopmental and growth impairment among extremely low-birth-weight infants with neonatal infection. JAMA, Vol.292, No.19 (Nov 17, 2004), pp. (2357-65), ISSN 1538-3598.

Sysmex Corporation. Operators Manual Sysmex XE-2100. 2005.

van der Meer, W., van Gelder, W., de Keijzer, R., & Willems, H. (2006). Does the band cell survive the 21st century? Eur J Haematol, Vol.76, No.3 (Mar, 2006), pp. (251-4), ISSN 0902-4441.

Vergnano, S., Sharland, M., Kazembe, P., Mwansambo, C., & Heath, P.T. (2005). Neonatal sepsis: an international perspective. Arch Dis Child Fetal Neonatal Ed, Vol.90, No.3 (May, 2005), pp. (F220-4), ISSN 1359-2998.

Weston, E.J., Pondo, T., Lewis, M.M., Martell-Cleary, P., Morin, C., Jewell, B., Daily, P., Apostol, M., Petit, S., Farley, M., Lynfield, R., Reingold, A., Hansen, N.I., Stoll, B.J., Shane, A.J., Zell, E., & Schrag, S.J. (2011). The burden of invasive early-onset neonatal sepsis in the United States, 2005-2008. Pediatr Infect Dis J, Vol.30, No.11 (Nov, 2011), pp. (937-41), ISSN 1532-0987.

Wirbelauer, J., Thomas, W., Rieger, L., & Speer, C.P. (2010). Intrauterine growth retardation in preterm infants </=32 weeks of gestation is associated with low white blood cell counts. Am J Perinatol, Vol.27, No.10 (Nov, 2010), pp. (819-24), ISSN 1098-8785.

Section 3

Prevention and Treatment

Chapter 6

Immunoglobulins in the Prevention and Treatment of Neonatal Sepsis

Elisabeth Resch and Bernhard Resch

Additional information is available at the end of the chapter

http://dx.doi.org/10.5772/54538

1. Introduction

It is a daily challenge and the most common clinical practise to rule out possible bacterial infection in the ill neonate and especially in the preterm infant. Approximately half of all newborn infants admitted to the neonatal ward carry a diagnosis of "rule-out sepsis", and diagnosis is often difficult as symptoms and signs of bacterial infection are subtle and nonspecific (1). The incidence of infection is higher in the neonatal period than at any other time of life, and factors that determine this increased susceptibility to bacterial infection include on the one hand the immaturity of the immune system with poor humoral responses to organisms (IgG and A), relatively poor neutrophil responses and complement activity, impaired macrophage function, and relatively poor T cell function, and on the other hand the exposure to microorganism from the maternal genital tract by ascending infections via the amniotic fluid or transplacental haematogenous spread. Additionally peripartum factors like trauma to skin or vessels during parturition or exposure to invasive obstetric procedures as well as portals of colonization and subsequent invasion (umbilicus, mucosal surfaces, eye, skin especially in very preterm infants) contribute to this increased risk for bacterial infection (2). Among extremely low birth weight infants at least 65% had one or more infections during their hospitalization in a National Institute of Child Health and Human Development Neonatal Research Network study including 6093 infants with follow-up at 18 to 22 months of corrected gestational age. Compared with uninfected infants infected infants were significantly more likely to have adverse neurodevelopmental outcomes at follow-up, including cerebral palsy (range of significant odds ratios [ORs], 1.4-1.7), low Bayley Scales of Infant Development II scores on the mental development index (ORs, 1.3-1.6) and psychomotor development index (ORs, 1.5-2.4), and vision impairment (ORs, 1.3-2.2). Infection in the neonatal period was also associated with impaired head growth, a known predictor of poor neurodevelopmental outcome (3). Reasons for the greater susceptibility to infection of preterm infants also include invasive procedures during their stay at the NICU, prolonged artificial ventilation, intravenous feeding and antibiotic pressures. (2). The incidence is estimated to range from 1 to 5-8.1 per 1000 live births (2,4). The proportion of child deaths that occurs in the neonatal period (38% in the year 2000) is increasing, and the Millennium Development Goal for child survival cannot be met without substantial reductions in neonatal mortality. Every year an estimated 4 million babies die in the first four weeks of life (the neonatal period), and, globally, the main direct causes of neonatal death are estimated to be preterm birth (28%), severe infections (26%), and asphyxia (23%) (5).

2. Pathophysiology of neonatal sepsis

The immune system of the neonate is immature in both humoral and cell mediated defense with prematurity further increasing the physiological inadequacies of the immune system. Sepsis spreads easily to the various organ systems in the neonates and thus, often presents as a multiorgan dysfunctions syndrome. Infection initiates a complex immune process, which includes antigen detection, T-cell activation and proliferation, and release of cytokines. Cytokines are low molecular mass proteins, which mediate cell growth, inflammation, immunity, differentiation, migration and repair. They regulate the amplitude and the duration of the inflammatory response and include interleukins-6 and -8, interferons-γ, colony-stimulating factors, tumour necrosis factor-α and others. However in the setting of overwhelming sepsis as a result to the microbial insult, these cytokines give rise to what is described as the systemic inflammatory response syndrome, where the much of the damage paradoxically results from the host defences (e.g. cytokines) analogous to a chain reaction themselves. The neutrophil functions: adhesion, diapedesis, phagocytosis and degranulation are also of prime importance in the host defence mechanisms against bacterial and fungal pathogens. The proteolytic enzymes released by the neutrophils are also damaging to the host tissue. Thus, immunoglobulins and neutrophils are responsible for both host defence and damage in the setting of overwhelming neonatal sepsis (6).

In 2005, definitions for paediatric infection, systemic inflammatory response syndrome, sepsis, severe sepsis, septic shock, and organ dysfunction were published that included term neonates of 0 to 7 days and newborns of 1 to 4 weeks of age (7). But one has to question why there are no criteria for the definition of sepsis and septic shock in preterm infants? The challenge of diagnosis of sepsis in the preterm infants is strongly associated with the immaturity of organ systems and transitional physiology. Suggested modifications of these definitions have recently been published (8) but still have to be proven in clinical trials (9).

3. Immunoglobulins and the innate immune response

Humoral immunity of the human newborn is provided primarily by maternal immunoglobulin G (IgG) transferred transplacentally, beginning at 8 to 10 weeks of gestation and accelerating during the last trimester. In a study to evaluate the role of maternally acquired antibody to native type III polysaccharide of group B *Streptococcus* as a determinant of susceptibility for infant systemic infection the authors found a significant correlation with maternal antibody levels in 111 acutely ill infants (10). These data extended earlier observations suggesting the correlation between low levels of type-specific antibody in serum and risk for systemic infection in neonates. Premature infants, compared to full-term infants, have lower levels of IgG at birth that further decreases during the first few weeks of life (11). The relative deficiency of humoral immunity in premature newborns might contribute to the inverse correlation of birth weight and rate of neonatal sepsis, with an 86-fold increased rate of sepsis in newborns of birth weight 600 to 999 grams compared to newborns of birth weight of more than 2500 grams (11). Ballow et al. (12) measured plasma immunoglobulin concentrations of premature infants of birth weight less than 1500 g longitudinally from birth to 10 months chronological age. During the first week of life plasma IgG levels correlated well with gestational age. At the age of three months mean plasma IgG levels were 60 mg/dl in infants of 25 to 28 weeks gestational age and 104 mg/dl in those of 29 to 32 weeks. Most infants remained hypogammaglobulinaemic at six months with 64% and 62%, respectively, of the infants having plasma IgG levels below 200 mg/dl. Plasma IgM concentrations were low in both groups during the first week of life (7.6 and 9.1 mg/dl, respectively) and rose to 41.8 and 34.7 mg/dl, respectively, by eight to ten months of life. IgA concentrations were comparable for both groups during the first week of life (1.2 and 0.6 mg/dl, respectively). After discharge Ballow et al. (12) followed 43 preterm infants until ten months chronological age and observed a significantly higher incidence of infections compared to 41 term infants ($p = 0.04$). In another study the level of maternal antibody required to protect neonates against early-onset disease caused by goup-B streptococci (GBS) type Ia was estimated (15). Levels of maternal serum IgG GBS Ia antibodies of 45 neonates with early onset disease case caused by GBS Ia and 319 control subjects (neonates colonized by GBS Ia but without early-onset disease) born at ≥34 weeks gestation were compared. The probability of developing infection declined with increasing maternal levels of IgG GBS Ia antibody ($P < .03$). Neonates whose mothers had levels of IgG GBS Ia antibody ≥5 mg/mL had an 88% lower risk (95% confidence interval, 7%–98%) of developing type-specific early-onset disease, compared with those whose mothers had levels <0.5 mg/mL (13).

Yang et al. (14) studied the mechanism of bacterial opsonization by intravenous immune globulin (IVIG) complement consumption and polymorphonuclear leukocyte membrane receptor mediated phagocytosis of Staphylococcus epidermidis, Klebsiella pneumoniae, and groups A and B streptococci. IGIV alone did not consume complement and showed no opsonic activity by itself for these organisms. When these bacteria were preopsonized in intravenous immune globulin, significant amounts of complement were consumed (44%-94%) and the uptake and killing of bacteria occurred. An important finding was the fact that in vitro opsonic activity of IGIV for these organisms was significantly correlated with the amount of complement consumed by the IVIG – opsonised bacteria. The in vivo protective efficacy of IVIG also appeared to be directly associated with its ability to activate and consume complement. The higher the titers of the IVIG preparation are (higher than 200 units:ml) the more opsonic activity has been shown towards slime-producing *S. epidermidis* (15). Administered as a prophylactic agent to low-birth weight (lower than 1700 g) preterm neonates immediately after birth revealed significantly higher specific IgG in blood sera compared to controls with an effect even lasting ten days after the last infusion. These results suggest that specific IgG titers might be well indicative of its opsonic activity against slime-producing *S. epidermidis* and might protect against bacteraemia.

The complement-inhibitory activity of different IVIG preparations was assessed in vitro by measurement of the blocking of C1q-, C4-, and C3 deposition on solid-phase aggregated rabbit IgG by enzyme-linked immunosorbent assay (16). Results showed that IgM enrichment of IVIG preparations enhances their effect to prevent the inflammatory effects of complement activation. No IgG preparation negatively affected in vitro phagocytosis of Escherichia coli by human granulocytes.

The mechanisms and effects of IVIGs are summarized in table 1 according to the description of Ballow (17).

- Fc receptor blockade of reticulo-endothelial cell system and mononuclear phagocytes
  - Competitive interaction of IVIG with anti-platelet antibodies for FC receptor
  - Soluble Fcγ receptors compete with membrane Fc receptors of the reticulo-endothelial system
- Modulation of Fc receptor expression or affinity
- Immunomodulation
  - Enhancement of T cell suppressor function
  - Inhibit B cell function and/or antigen-processing cells via Fc receptor
- Restoration of idiotype-antiidiotypic network
- Modify complement-dependent immune damage to tissue and cells
- Inhibit cytokine/interleukin production/action
- "Neutralize" toxin superantigen
- Soluble CD4 and CD8, soluble HLA Class II molecules that modulate antigen processing and/or T cell activation

Table 1. Mechanisms of action of intravenous immune globulins (17)

Similar to most immunoglobins, the transplacental transport of IgG from the mother to fetus begins around 32 weeks of gestational age and increases until term. Premature infants born prior to 32 weeks gestation have profound IgG deficiencies. The major function of IgG in host defense is to opsonize bacteria and neutralize viruses. Levels of postnatal IgG are often low due to insufficient production by the immature neonatal immune system and catabolism of maternal IgG. Opsonic activity is also type-specific; therefore humoral immunity transferred to the neonate will be insufficient if the mother does not have immunity to the specific pathogen (18).

4. Immunoglobulins in neonates

Immunotherapy was a common method of treatment of infectious diseases in the preantibiotic era with serotherapy being a popular approach to serious infections by use of antisera from large animals. This administration unfortunately was associated with the risk of anaphylaxis and serum sickness. Further on immune globulins obtained from pooled human plasma were used, but antibodies provided by these preparations always represented those common to the donor population, and intravenous injection of early human IgG preparations was complicated by severe allergic reactions (19). The next step was the purification of human immune globulins, and, currently there are multiple formulations of safe, pooled, human immunoglobulins tor the intravenous use.

The mortality rate of the preterm infants with septicaemia decreased from 44% in the infants receiving only antibiotics to 8% in the infants treated by IVIG together with the same antibiotic following administration of IVIG to preterm neonates (0.3 g/day in neonates below 1000 g; 0.5 g/day in neonates over 1000 g for 6 consecutive days). The IVIG preparation was well-tolerated by all newborns, and no adverse events were observed by monitoring blood gas analysis, clinical examination, monitoring of respiration, pulse and body temperature. Follow-up at an average age of 2.5 years showed no evidence of harmful effects of IVIG treatment in the neonatal period (20).

Cates et al. (21) evaluated the formation of specific and functional antibody in preterm infants born weighing less than 1500 g (mean 1088 g) and less than 32 weeks of gestational age (mean 28.8 weeks). In the presence of complement, the strain of coagulase negative staphylococcus used was opsonized by IgG antibody, and the strain of Escherichia coli by IgM. Geometric mean plasma levels of tetanus and diphtheria IgG antibody fell from birth to 4 months chronological age, but rose significantly by 9 months (approximately 2 months after the third dose of diphtheria, tetanus, pertussis vaccine). However, at 9 months they remained lower than the respective geometric mean levels in 9-month-old term infants. The preterm infants' mean plasma IgG staphylococcal opsonic activity fell from birth to 2.5 months, but by 9 months was comparable to that of term infants of the same age. Mean IgM opsonic activity for Escherichia coli was very low at birth in both preterm and term infants. It rose with chronological age, correlating with the rise in total IgM by 9 months the mean preterm and term infants' levels of IgM opsonic activity for E. coli were comparable.

Sasidharan (22) studied serially IgG levels postnatally in 42 infants of very low birth weight with gestational ages ranging from 23 to 31 weeks (mean birth weight 971 g). Eighteen infants (43%) had IgG levels of less than 100 mg/dl by a mean postnatal age of 71 days. The lowest level was found in a 700g infant with 22 mg/dl. In sixteen cases having cord blood IgG levels determined mean IgG values was 414 mg/dl. This had dropped to a mean of 140 mg/dl by 57 days. As expected, the lowest IgG levels postnatally were a reflection of the degree of prematurity and the length of postnatal age.

To proof the significance of low serum IgG and complement proteins in very low birth neonates Lassiter et al (23) measured serum IgG, C3, C4 and Factor B weekly by rate nephelometry in 15 neonates who developed proven nosocomial bacterial or candidal sepsis and 27 neonates who did not develop sepsis. In the first and second week of life the serum IgG of infected neonates was significantly lower (mean 295 and 270 mg/dl compared to 440 and 473 mg/dl, respectively. If the IgG was less than 350 mg/dl in the first week or less than 230 mg/dl in the second week, the relative risk of acquiring sepsis was greater than or equal to 5 (CI 95% 1.7 to 11.2).

Amato et al. (24) investigated serial IgG and IgM serum levels during the neonatal period in two groups of non-septic, preterm infants treated prophylactic with IVIG. Twenty-two very low birth weight infants (mean gestational age 31.8 weeks and mean birth weight 1265 g with a range of 1001 - 1500g) and 12 extremely low birth weight infants < 1000g (mean gestational age 28.6 weeks and mean birth weight 910g) received at random three standard doses of IVIG (0.5 g/kg/day) or IVIGAM (IgM enriched preparation) (5 ml/kg/day). IgG and IgM concentrations were assayed by rate nephelometry before treatment and at day 3, 5, 7, 14 and 28 of life. At any time IgG levels were higher in the IVIG very low birth weight group and no difference was observed in the extremely low birth weight group. IgM levels were higher at day 3 and 5 in the IVIGAM very low birth weight group and until day 7 in the extremely low birth weight group. The authors concluded that their findings indicate a wide range of IgG and IgM kinetics in the healthy premature infant.

Supplementation of the preterm serum with either intravenous immunoglobulin or IgM-enriched immunoglobulin did not change the results of phagocytosis rates (percentage of neutrophils phagocytosing group B streptococci in vitro in infants < 32 weeks of gestation and adult controls) significantly (25).

In a rat model marked neutropenia, complete depletion of the neutrophil storage pool, and death within 48 hours were observed in newborn rats intrapulmonically inoculated with type III group B streptococci (26). Intraperitoneal administration of 225 mg of IVIG immediately after intrapulmonic inoculation of GBS significantly lessened the degree of neutropenia and prevented depletion of the neutrophil storage pool and death. No effect of IVIG on neutrophil production was observed in vitro or in vivo in normal neonatal rats injected with IVIG. IVIG, however, markedly hastened release of neutrophils from the reserves into the blood and hastened the arrival of neutrophils at the site of the bacterial injection. Specific antibody to GBS, as opposed to a nonspecific IgG effect, appeared to be responsible for the improvements in neutrophils kinetics and for survival of the animals.

In animal experiments following administration of IVIGAM endotoxemia was induced by intraperitoneal inoculation of a sublethal dose of Escherichia coli and subsequent intravenous administration of an antimicrobial agent (27). Prophylactic administration of IVIGAM was found to significantly attenuate the antibiotic-induced increase in endotoxin activity as compared to the albumin control group. These experimental results suggested that in endotoxaemia the polyclonal immunoglobulin preparation had a prophylactic protective effect on the acute phase responses and reduced the cardiodepressant effects of Escherichia coli septicaemia.

The pharmacokinetics and safety of IVIG were examined in thirty neonates with suspected sepsis who were randomly assigned either to a treatment (receiving either 250, or 500, or 1,000 mg/kg of IVIG plus antibiotics) or control (antibiotics alone) group (28). The 500 mg/kg dose produced a rise in total IgG for greater than 8 and in group B streptococcus type-specific IgG for greater than 4-14 days. The type-specific antibody elevation varied with the amount of pathogen-specific antibody and dose of IVIG. Pharmacokinetic analysis suggested a biphasic elimination curve and a terminal elimination half-life of 24.2 days. No toxicity was observed (28).

Prophylactic IVIG at a dose of 0.5 g/kg/day was given prospectively in 28 healthy preterm infants with a mean gestational age of 29.4 weeks and weight of 1,387g when they were 3-10 days old (29). Urine samples of the neonates were obtained for analysis on days 1, 2 and 3 following IVIG administration as well as 1 day before; and urinary nitrite levels were 2.77 +/- 1.66 μmol/mmol creatinine before IVIG administration; 4.33 +/- 3.88 μmol/mmol creatinine on the 1st; 3.77 +/- 2.73 μmol/mmol creatinine on the 2nd, and 3.64 +/- 3.28 μmol/mmol creatinine on the 3rd day. The increase of urinary nitrite levels was significant between before and after IVIG administration, thereafter levels did not differ significantly, suggesting that endogenous NO formation might play an important role in both the therapeutic and adverse effects of IVIG (29).

5. Use of immunoglobulins in the treatment of neonatal sepsis

Polyvalent immunoglobulin preparations are widely used as adjunctive therapy for sepsis or septic shock, but their efficacy is still a matter of debate. In 2007 Kreymann et al. (30) conducted a systematic review summarizing data on adults and neonates separately. In neonates, 12 trials (31-42) involving 710 patients were published. The estimate of the pooled effect on mortality was RR = 0.56 (95% CI 0.42– 0.74, p <.0001). Five studies (32,35,37,39,41) involving 352 patients were performed with the IgGAM preparation. The range of the cumulative dose of IgG was 0.57– 0.76 g/kg birth weight plus 0.09–0.12 g/kg birth weight IgA and 0.09–0.12 g/kg birth weight IgM. In this subgroup, the estimate of the pooled effect was RR = 0.50 (95% CI 0.34–0.73), equivalent to a 50% relative reduction in mortality ($p <$ .0003). The study effects were comparable, and the test of heterogeneity was not significant. The study of El Nawawy (32) reported a significant reduction of mortality, the other four a positive trend (35,37,39,41). Polyvalent immunoglobulin preparations containing only IgG were evaluated in seven trials (31,33,34,36,38,40,42) involving 358 patients. The cumulative dose of IgG was 0.5–3 g/kg birth weight. The estimate of the pooled effect for this subgroup was RR = 0.63 (95% CI 0.42– 0.96), equivalent to a 37% relative reduction in mortality (p < .03). The test of heterogeneity was not significant. One study (38) reported a significant reduction in mortality, three studies reported a positive trend (31,33,42), and two studies (34,40) showed no effect. One trial (36) showed a duplication of mortality; one neonate died in the control group and two in the treatment group. Comparing the two treatment modalities, a small and insignificant difference in favour of IgGAM was observed (z = 0.80, p ≤ .42). Kreymann et al. (30) found a negative correlation with the severity of illness (as measured by the mortality of the control groups) in neonates; however, this held true only when the results reported by Chen (36) were included: In this study, an exceptionally low mortality in the control group was observed (1 of 28, respectively, 3.6%), which was doubled in the treatment group (2 of 28, respectively, 7.1%). If these results were omitted, the correlation lost significance. Additionally the authors found no correlation with the dosage of immunoglobulins administered.

In adults and children, Kreymann et al. (30) found a strong trend in favour of IgGAM over IgG preparations with a 34% and 15% reduction of the risk to die, respectively, compared to an even higher 50% and 37% relative reduction of mortality in neonates, respectively. In neonates and especially preterm infants, therapy with polyclonal immunoglobulins should be understood much more as a substitutional therapy than as an adjunctive therapy as for adults or older children (43). Comparing the two treatment modalities (IgGAM vs. IgG) in neonates, Kreymann et al. (30) only found a slight difference without statistical significance. A major limitation of this meta-analysis is the inclusion of the study of El Nawawy (32), who originally included infants of 1 to 24 months of age hospitalized at a pediatric intensive care unit, of which 50 were proven septic patients. This study strongly influenced study results favouring immunoglobulin therapy.

Ohlsson and Lacy (44) recently reviewed IVIG for suspected or subsequently proven infection in neonates including randomized or quasi-randomized controlled trials comparing IVIG treatment to placebo or no intervention in newborn infants below 28 days of age. They found 10 studies meeting their inclusion criteria that differed to the above mentioned analysis (30) by additional including the small study of Christensen et al. (45) and a new study by Ahmend et al. (46) and not including the studies by El Nawawy (32), Gökalp (38), and Gunes (31).The results showed a statistically significant reduction in mortality in cases of proven and also of suspected infection with a NNT of 10 infants (95% CI; 6, 33) to avoid one death.

IVIG preparations with high concentrations of antibodies to bacteria that are commonly isolated from neonates in specific local settings or geographical areas may be more effective in reducing adverse outcomes (44). However, the use of antistaphylococcal immunoglobulins to prevent staphylococcal infection in very low birth weight infants has recently been reviewed and is currently not recommended (47).

A very recent study published by the International Neonatal Immunotherapy Study (INIS) Collaborative group enrolled 3493 infants with birth weight less than 1500g receiving antibiotics for suspected or proven serious infection and randomly assigned them to receive two infusions of either IgG immune globulin (at a dose of 500 mg per kilogram of body weight) or matching placebo 48 hours apart (48). The researchers found no significant between-group difference in the rates of death or major disability at the age of two years (39 and 39%, respectively). Similarly, there were no significant differences in the rates of secondary outcomes including the incidence of subsequent sepsis episodes. In the 2-years follow-up of the study participants there were no differences in the rates of major or non-major disability or of adverse events. Thus, IgG IVIG was not found to be helpful in diminishing the risk of major complications or adverse outcomes in neonates with suspected or proven sepsis. The duration of hospital stay also did not differ between groups (48).

The clinical efficacy of IgM-enriched IVIG (currently there is only one preparation available, Pentaglobin®) has been reviewed by Norrby-Teglund et al. (49) for both adult and paediatric/neonatal patients. The authors concluded that patients most likely to benefit are Gram-negative septic shock patients. Therefore it is important to emphasize that selection of study patients as well as microbiological aetiology are of high relevance affecting the efficacy of IVIG.

6. Use of immunoglobulins in the prevention of neonatal sepsis

There have been published a lot of studies and reviews on the preventive use of IVIG in preterm infants and I herewith report ("pars pro toto") two multicenter randomized, double-blind, placebo-controlled trial published early in the New England Journal of Medicine (50,51) with divergent results and the latest Cochrane Review (52).

Baker et al. (50) included 588 infants with a birth weight of 500 - 1750 g and age of 3 - 7 days from six centres in the U.S. between 1987 and 1988. The trial was randomized, double-blind, placebo-controlled with 287 infants having received 500 mg/kg of IVIG at enrolment (age 3 to 7 days), one week later, and then every 14 days until a total of five infusions had been given or until hospital discharge, whichever came first, and 297 controls having received an equal volume of a sterile solution of 5 % albumin and 0.9 % sodium chloride. Outcomes included proven infection - clinical findings of sepsis and at least one of the following: a positive blood culture of either bacteria or fungi (the isolation of a pathogen from a normally sterile other body site or urine obtained by suprapubic or bladder catheterization, or the isolation of virus from an infant with clinical deterioration), necrotizing enterocolitis stage II or III, intraventricular haemorrhage grade 1 to 4, bronchopulmonary dysplasia, death, and total days in hospital. There were 50 episodes of sepsis among 287 infants (17.4%) in the IVIG group and 75 episodes of sepsis among 297 infants (25.3%) in the placebo group. The cumulative relative risk reduction was 0.7 (CI 95% 0.5-0.9).

In a prospective, multicenter, two-phase controlled trial, Fanaroff et al. (51) stratified 2416 infants according to birth weight (501 to 1000 g and 1001 to 1500 g) and randomly assigned to an IVIG (n = 1204) or a control group (n = 1212). Control infants were given placebo infusions during phase 1 of the study (n = 623) but were not given any infusions during phase 2 (n = 589). Infants weighing 501 to 1000 g at birth were given 900 mg of immune globulin per kilogram of body weight, and infants weighing 1001 to 1500 g at birth were given a dose of 700 mg per kilogram. The immune globulin infusions were repeated every 14 days until the infants weighed 1800 g, were transferred to another center, died, or were sent home from the hospital. Nosocomial infections of the blood, meninges, or urinary tract occurred in 439 of the 2416 infants (18.2 %): 208 (17.3 %) in the immune globulin group and 231 (19.1%) in the control group (relative risk, 0.91; CI 95% 0.77 to 1.08). Septicemia occurred in 15.5% of the immune globulin recipients and 17.2% of the controls. The predominant organisms included gram-positive cocci (53%), gram-negative bacilli (22.4%), and candida species (16%). Adverse reactions were rarely observed during the infusions. Immune globulin therapy had no effect on respiratory distress syndrome, bronchopulmonary dysplasia, intracranial hemorrhage, the duration of hospitalization, or mortality. The incidence of necrotizing enterocolitis was 12% in the immune globulin group and 9.5" in the control group. Thus, the authors concluded that the prophylactic use of IVIG failed to reduce the incidence of hospital-acquired infections in very-low-birth-weight infants (51).

The prophylactic administration of intravenous immunoglobulins (IVIG) to prevent nosocomial infections has been studied in >5,000 neonates from 19 studies enrolled in randomised controlled trials (52). The results of these meta-analyses showed a statistically significant reduction in sepsis (number needed to treat – NNT - 36) and/or any serious infection (NNT 31), but no reduction in mortality from infection. The reviewers concluded that IVIG administration resulted in a 3% reduction in sepsis and a 4% reduction in any serious infection of one or more episodes. Nevertheless it was not associated with reductions in other important outcomes including necrotizing enterocolitis intraventricular haemorrhage, or length of hospital stay. Most importantly, IVIG administration did not have any significant effect on mortality from any cause or from infections. There were no adverse events observed to be associated with prophylactic use of IVIG. From a clinical perspective a 3-4% reduction in nosocomial infections without a reduction in mortality or other important clinical outcomes might be of marginal importance and has to be outweighed by the costs and the values assigned to the clinical outcomes (52). This Cochrane review ends with the statement that there is no justification for further randomized trials testing the efficacy of previously studied IVIG preparations to reduce nosocomial infections in preterm and/or low birth weight infants. In contrast, these results should encourage basic scientists and clinicians to pursue other avenues to prevent nosocomial infections (52).

7. Conclusions

There is a rational to use of IVIG in either adjunctive treatment neonatal sepsis or in the prevention by low immunoglobulin levels associated with the immature innate immune system of preterm infants. Studies so far revealed a benefit for IgM enriched IVIG in the use as adjunctive sepsis treatment by an overall significantly reduced mortality rate. Prophylactic use of IVIG resulted in marginally reduced rates of nosocomial infections, and other non-invasive approaches like use of lactoferrin (53) and/or probiotics (54) seem to be more promising in the prevention of nosocomial infections in very low birth weight infants.

Author details

Elisabeth Resch and Bernhard Resch
Research Unit for Neonatal Infectious Diseases and Epidemiology, Division of Neonatology, Department of Pediatrics, Medical University of Graz, Austria

8. References

[1] Escobar GJ. The neonatal "sepsis work-up": personal reflections on the development of an evidence-based approach toward newborn infections in a managed care organization. Pediatrics 1999;103:360–733.
[2] Issacs D, Moxon ER. Handbook of neonatal infections, a practical guide. WB Saunders, London, Edinburgh, New York, Philadelphia, Sydney, Tokio1999, pp1-13
[3] Stoll BJ, Hansen NI, Adams-Chapman I, Fanaroff AA, Hintz SR, Vohr B, Higgins RD; National Institute of Child Health and Human Development Neonatal Research

Network. Neurodevelopmental and growth impairment among extremely low-birth-weight infants with neonatal infection. JAMA 2004;292:2357-2365.
[4] Gerdes JS. Diagnosis and management of bacterial infections in the neonate. Pediatr Clin North Am 2004;51:939-959
[5] Lawn JE, Cousens S, Zupan J; Lancet Neonatal Survival Steering Team. 4 million neonatal deaths: when? Where? Why? Lancet 2005;365:891-900.
[6] Shaw CK, Thapalial A, Shaw P, Malla K. Intravenous immunoglobulins and haematopoietic growth factors in the prevention and treatment of neonatal sepsis: ground reality or glorified myths? Int J Clin Pract 2007;61:482–487
[7] Goldstein B, Giroir B, Randolph A. International pediatric sepsis consensus conference: definitions for sepsis and organ dysfunction in pediatrics. Pediatr Crit Care Med 2005;6:2-8.
[8] Wynn JL, Wong HR. Pathophysiology and treatment of septic shock in neonates. Clin Perinatol 2010;37:439-479
[9] Hofer N, Zacharias E, Müller W, Resch B. Performance of the definitions of the systemic inflammatory response syndrome and sepsis in neonates. J Perinat Med 2012 Jun 14;0(0):1-4. doi: 10.1515/jpm-2011-0308.
[10] Baker CJ, Edwards MD, Kasper DL. Role of Antibody to Native Type III Polysaccharide of Group B Streptococcus in Infant Infection. Pediatrics 1981;68:544 -549
[11] Jenson HB, Pollock BH. Meta-analyses of the Effectiveness of Intravenous Immune Globulin for Prevention and Treatment of Neonatal Sepsis. Pediatrics 1997;99: e2 doi: 10.1542/peds.99.2.e2
[12] Ballow M, Cates KL, Rowe JC, Goetz C, Desbonnet C. Development of the immune system in very low birth weight (less than 1500 g) premature infants: concentrations of plasma immunoglobulins and patterns of infections. Pediatr Res 1986;20:899-904.
[13] Lin FYC, Philips III JB, Azimi PH, Weisman LE, Clark P, Rhoads GG, Regan J, Concepcion NF, Frasch CE, Troendle J, Brenner RA, Gray BM, Bhushan, Fitzgerald G, Moye P, Clemens JD. Level of maternal antibody required to protect neonates against early-onset disease caused by group b streptococcus type Ia: a multicenter, seroepidemiology study. J Infect Dis 2001;184:1022–1028
[14] Yang KD, Bathras JM, Shigeoka AO, James J, Pincus SH, Hill HR. Mechanisms of bacterial opsonization by immune globulin intravenous: correlation of complement consumption with opsonic activity and protective efficacy. J Infect Dis 1989;159:701-707
[15] Lamari F. Determination of slime-producing S. epidermidis specific antibodies in human immunoglobulin preparations and blood sera by an enzyme immunoassay. Correlation of antibody titers with opsonic activity and application to preterm neonates. J Pharm Biomed Ana 2000;23:363–374
[16] Rieben R, Roos A, Muizert Y, Tinguely C, Gerritsen AF, Daha MR. Immunoglobulin M-Enriched Human Intravenous Immunoglobulin Prevents Complement Activation In Vitro and In Vivo in a Rat Model of Acute Inflammation. Blood 1999 93: 942-951
[17] Ballow M. Mechanisms of action of intravenous immune serum globulin therapy. Pediatr Infect Dis J 1994;13:806-811

[18] Melvan JN, Bagby GJ, Welsh DA, Nelson S, Zhang P. Neonatal Sepsis and Neutrophil Insufficiencies. Int Rev Immunol. 2010; 29: 315–348

[19] Kliegman RM, Clapp DW. Rational principles for immunoglobulin prophylaxis and therapy of neonatal infections. Clin Perinatol 1991;18:303-324.

[20] von Muralt G, Sidiropoulos D. Prenatal and postnatal prophylaxis of infections in preterm neonates. Pediatr Infect Dis J 1988;7(5 Suppl):S72-78.

[21] Cates KL, Goetz C, Rosenberg N, Pantschenko A, Rowe JC, Ballow M. Longitudinal development of specific and functional antibody in very low birth weight premature infants. Pediatr Res 1988;23:14-22.

[22] Sasidharan P. Postnatal IgG levels in very-low-birth-weight infants. Preliminary observations. Clin Pediatr (Phila) 1988;27:271-274.

[23] Lassiter HA, Tanner JE, Cost KM, Steger S, Vogel RL. Diminished IgG, but not complement C3 or C4 or factor B, precedes nosocomial bacterial sepsis in very low birth weight neonates. Pediatr Infect Dis J 1991;10:663-668.

[24] Amato M, Hüppi P, Imbach P, Llanto A, Bürgi W. Serial IgG and IgM serum levels after infusion of different Ig-preparations (IgG or IgM-enriched) in preterm infants. Pediatr Allergy Immunol. 1993 Nov;4(4):217-20.

[25] Bialek R, Bartmann P. Is there an effect of immunoglobulins and G-CSF on neutrophil phagocytic activity in preterm infants? Infection 1998;26:375-378.

[26] Redd H, Christensen RD, Fischer GW. Circulating and storage neutrophils in septic neonatal rats treated with immune globulin. J Infect Dis. 1988;157:705-712.

[27] Oesser S, Schulze C, Seifert J. Protective capacity of a IgM/IgA-enriched polyclonal immunoglobulin-G preparation in endotoxemia. Res Exp Med (Berl) 1999;198:325-339.

[28] Weisman LE, Fischer GW, Marinelli P, Hemming VG, Pierce JR, Golden SM, Peck CC. Pharmacokinetics of intravenous immunoglobulin in neonates. Vox Sang 1989;57:243-248.

[29] Özkan H, Uzuner N, Ören H, Çabuk N, Islekel H. Urinary nitrite excretion after prophylactic intravenous immunoglobulin in premature infants. Biol Neonate 2000;77:101-104

[30] Kreymann KG, de Heer G, Nierhaus A, Kluge S. Use of polyclonal immunoglobulins as adjunctive therapy for sepsis or septic shock. Crit Care Med 2007;35:2677-2685

[31] Gunes T, Koklu E, Buyukkayhan D, Kurtoglu S, Karakukcu M, Patiroglu T. Exchange transfusion or intravenous immunoglobulin therapy as an adjunct to antibiotics for neonatal sepsis in developing countries: A pilot study. Ann Trop Paediatr 2006; 26:39–42

[32] El Nawawy A, El Kinany H, Hamdy El-Sayed M, Boshra N. Intravenous polyclonal immunoglobulin administration to sepsis syndrome patients: A prospective study in a pediatric intensive care unit. J Trop Pediatr 2005; 51:271–278

[33] Weisman LE, Stoll BJ, Kueser TJ, Rubio TT, Frank CG, Heiman HS, Subramanian KN, Hankins CT, Anthony BF, Cruess DF, et al. Intravenous immune globulin therapy for early- onset sepsis in premature neonates. J Pediatr 1992; 121:434–443

[34] Shenoi A, Nagesh NK, Maiya PP, Bhat SR, Subba Rao SD. Multicenter randomized placebo controlled trial of therapy with intravenous immunoglobulin in decreasing mortality due to neonatal sepsis. Indian Pediatr 1999; 36:1113–1118

[35] Samantha S, Jalalu MP, Hegde RK, et al: Role of IgM enriched intravenous immunoglobulin as an adjuvant to antibiotics in neonatal sepsis. Karnataka Pediatr J 1997; 1:1–6

[36] Chen JY: Intravenous immunoglobulin in the treatment of full-term and premature newborns with sepsis. J Formos Med Assoc 1996; 95:839–844

[37] Seitz RC, Turreson M, Grosse R, et al: Infusion of immunoglobulins for therapy of neonatal sepsis. Z Geburtshilfe Perinatol 1995; 199:288

[38] Gökalp AS, Toksoy HB, Turkay S, Bakici MZ, Kaya R. Intravenous immunoglobulin in the treatment of Salmonella typhimurium infections in preterm neonates. Clin Pediatr (Phila) 1994; 33:349–352

[39] Erdem G, Yurdakok M, Tekinalp G, Ersoy F. The use of IgM-enriched intravenous immunoglobulin for the treatment of neonatal sepsis in preterm infants. Turk J Pediatr 1993; 35: 277–281

[40] Mancilla-Ramirez J, Gonzalez-Yunes R, Castellanos-Cruz C, García-Roca P, Santos-Preciado JI. Intravenous immunoglobulin in the treatment of neonatal septicemia. Bol Med Hosp Infant Mex 1992; 49:4–11

[41] Haque KN, Zaidi MH, Bahakim H: IgMenriched intravenous immunoglobulin therapy in neonatal sepsis. Am J Dis Child 1988; 142:1293–1296

[42] Sidiropoulos D, Böhme U, von Muralt G, Morell A, Barandun S. Substitution of immunoglobulins for the treatment of neonatal sepsis. Schweiz Med Wochenschr 1981; 111:1649–1655

[43] Bell SG: Immunomodulation, part III: Intravenous immunoglobulin. Neonatal Netw 2006; 25:213–221

[44] Ohlsson A, Lacy J. Intravenous immunoglobulin for suspected or subsequently proven infection in neonates. Cochrane Database of Systematic Reviews 2010, Issue 3. Art. No.: CD001239. DOI: 10.1002/14651858.CD001239.pub3.

[45] Christensen RD, Brown MS, Hall DC, Lassiter HA, Hill HR. Effect of neutrophil kinetics and serum opsonic capacity of intravenous administration of immune globulin to neonates with clinical signs of early-onset sepsis. Journal of Pediatrics 1991;118: 606–614.

[46] Ahmed SS, Chowdhury MAKA, Hoque MM, Begum D, Ahmed ASMNU. Role of intravenous immunoglobulin (IVIG) as an adjuvant in the treatment of neonatal sepsis in preterm babies. Journal of Bangladesh College of Physicians and Surgeons 2006;24:97–104.

[47] Shah PS, Kaufman DA. Antistaphyloccoccal immunoglobulins to prevent staphylococcal infection in very low birth weight infants. Cochrane Database of Systematic Reviews 2009, Issue 2. [DOI: 10.1002/14651858.CD006449.pub2]

[48] INIS Collaborative Group. Brocklehurst P, Farrell B, King A, Juszczak E, Darlow B, Haque K, Salt A, Stenson B, Tarnow-Mordi W. Treatment of neonatal sepsis with intravenous immune globulinN Engl J Med 2011;365:1201-1211.

[49] Norrby-Teglund A, Haque KN, L. Hammarström L. Intravenous polyclonal IgM-enriched immunoglobulin therapy in sepsis: a review of clinical efficacy in relation to microbiological aetiology and severity of sepsis. Journal of Internal Medicine 2006; 260: 509–516

[50] Baker CJ, Melish ME, Hall RT, et al. Intravenous immune globulin for the prevention of nosocomial infection in low-birth-weight neonates. New Engl JMed 1992;327:213–219.

[51] Fanaroff AA, Korones SB, Wright LL, Wright EC, Poland RL, Bauer CB, Tyson JE, Philips JB 3rd, Edwards W, Lucey JF, et al. A controlled trial of intravenous immune globulin to reduce nosocomial infections in very-low-birth-weight infants. National Institute of Child Health and Human Development Neonatal Research Network. New Engl J Med 1994;330(:1107-13.

[52] Ohlsson A, Lacy JB. Intravenous immunoglobulin for preventing infection in preterm and/or low-birth-weight infants. Cochrane Database Syst Rev 2004;(1):CD000361

[53] Manzoni P, Rinaldi M, Cattani S, Pugni L, Romeo MG, Messner H, Stolfi I, Decembrino L, Laforgia N, Vagnarelli F, Memo L, Bordignon L, Saia OS, Maule M, Gallo E, Mostert M, Magnani C, Quercia M, Bollani L, Pedicino R, Renzullo L, Betta P, Mosca F, Ferrari F, Magaldi R, Stronati M, Farina D; Italian Task Force for the Study and Prevention of Neonatal Fungal Infections, Italian Society of Neonatology. Bovine lactoferrin supplementation for prevention of late-onset sepsis in very low-birth-weight neonates: a randomized trial. JAMA 2009;302:1421-1428.

[54] Alfaleh K, Anabrees J, Bassler D, Al-Kharfi T. Probiotics for prevention of necrotizing enterocolitis in preterm infants. Cochrane Database Syst Rev 2011 Mar 16;(3):CD005496.